s' Aids Series

GERIATRIC NURSING

NURSES' AIDS SER

ANAESTHETICS FOR NURSES

ANATOMY AND PHYSIOLOGY FOR NURSES

ARITHMETIC IN NURSING

EAR, NOSE AND THROAT NURSING

GERIATRIC NURSING

MEDICAL NURSING

MICROBIOLOGY FOR NURSES

OBSTETRIC AND GYNAECOLOGICAL NURSING

OPHTHALMIC NURSING

ORTHOPAEDICS FOR NURSES

PAEDIATRIC NURSING

PERSONAL AND COMMUNITY HEALTH

PHARMACOLOGY FOR NURSES

PRACTICAL PROCEDURES

PSYCHIATRIC NURSING

PSYCHOLOGY FOR NURSES

SURGICAL NURSING

THEATRE TECHNIQUE

TROPICAL HYGIENE AND NURSING

Nurses' Aids Series

Geriatric Nursing

Alison M. F. Storrs
SRN, SCM
Ward Sister, Geriatric Unit, Pembury Hospital, Tunbridge Wells

BAILLIÈRE TINDALL LONDON

a division of
Cassell & Collier Macmillan Publishers Ltd., London
34 Red Lion Square, London WC1R 4SG
Sydney, Auckland, Toronto, Johannesburg

Macmillan Publishing Company
New York

First published 1976
Reprinted 1978
ISBN 0 7020 0580 0

Printed by Cox & Wyman Ltd,
London, Fakenham and Reading

Preface

This book is written for the benefit of student and pupil nurses, especially those undergoing their secondment to a geriatric unit. It should also be useful to those registered and enrolled nurses who undertake the course approved by the Joint Board of Clinical Studies and to all nurses working in the community. In addition, I hope it will be of interest to nurses in the fields of general medicine, surgery and orthopaedics, who are often dealing with elderly patients.

The book covers all aspects of the care required by the geriatric patient in hospital and during rehabilitation at the day hospital. It describes the place of the geriatric unit in relation to the community and hospital services, and emphasizes the importance of team work and the role of the geriatric nurse within that team. She is one of the most important members, spending the most time with the patient, beginning the rehabilitation process on the patient's admission to hospital and continuing that process throughout the patient's stay. Upon her depends the success or failure of the patient's visit. So, although good nursing care is learned on the ward and not from books, the text includes wherever possible practical guidance and detail on assisting the patient to overcome the difficulties which hinder rehabilitation and to achieve maximum mobility and independence. The chapters on bedsores and incontinence, two demanding aspects of geriatric care, are examples of this approach.

The nurse also needs to extend her skills in the rehabilitation field itself, so that she can work closely with the physiotherapist, occupational therapist and speech therapist, carrying on some of the work which they have begun. The role of the nurse in the geriatric unit is exciting and imaginative for all those willing to accept the opportunities it provides.

Throughout the text the patient has been referred to as 'he' and the nurse as 'she' purely for the sake of clarity.

I wish to thank Dr C. W. J. Ussher, Consultant Physician in Geriatric Medicine to the Tunbridge Wells Health District, for writing the first two chapters and for his criticism and help with the remainder of the book; the staff of the Geriatric Unit of Pembury Hospital for their help and encouragement; Leonard Warner for the line drawings; and Peter Broadbury and Trevor Hill, of the Department of Medical Illustration, Queen Victoria Hospital, East Grinstead, for the photographs. I also owe acknowledgement to Dr Trevor Howells for Figs. 2 and 3, and to Professor Bernard Isaacs for Fig. 12. Finally, my thanks to my publishers, Baillière Tindall, for their assistance throughout the preparation of the book.

September 1975 A. STORRS

Contents

List of Plates

The following illustrations appear between pages 120 and 121

1 An Introduction to Geriatrics

To those working in this field for the first time some of the terms used can be confusing, and it may be helpful to start with some definitions.

The word *geriatric* is derived from the Greek *geron* meaning an old man and *iatros* meaning a doctor. Unfortunately the word is nowadays used very loosely as either a noun or an adjective, but it has undoubtedly come to stay. Geriatrics may be defined as the branch of general medicine concerned with the clinical, social, preventive and remedial aspects of illness in the elderly.

Gerontology is the study of ageing, which is a normal process; a great deal of research is carried out in centres all over the world, particularly Baltimore and Kiev. The derogatory words *senile* and *senility*, implying feebleness and that nothing can be done, are best avoided except in reference to dementia, which is a specific form of insanity consisting of feebleness rather than derangement and especially common in old age. A better word for the ageing process is *senescence*, which begins in our twenties when we cease growing and continues relentlessly throughout our life span.

Two other words frequently used in the practice of geriatrics are disablement (or disability) and rehabilitation. *Disablement* is any handicap of a permanent or temporary nature caused by physical, sensory or mental affliction or any defect which prevents a person living a full life as a human being and makes him a burden to himself, his environment or his society. *Rehabilitation* is any systematic activity which helps a person to overcome or diminish disablement and to minimize its social consequences.

The Ageing Process

Old age is not a disease in the true sense of the word, but is a retrograde biological change which leads to decreased powers of survival and adjustment. The rate of this process varies from individual to individual, from organ to organ and even from cell type to cell type. Individual differences arise not only from heredity, but also from the environment and the ravages of life both physical and mental. This process occurs in all of us after we reach the peak of growth in our early twenties. From this time on the states of 'active growth' and 'involution' vary as we grow older. The degenerative processes gradually take over and continue at a faster rate than active growth. Nonetheless, active growth does continue to some degree through our life span—injuries heal, blood cells are replaced and the heart will hypertrophy in hypertension.

Outward appearance The tendency with age is to grow lighter and become smaller in build. The posture is that of flexion, with the head held forward, the spine bowed and the hips and knees flexed. The loss of height is aggravated by muscular weakness, joint degeneration and osteoporosis. The face becomes shrunken and wrinkled as subcutaneous fat is lost and the jaw bones atrophy due to the edentulous state. Loss of elasticity in the skin makes it difficult to assess clinically the state of hydration. The hair tends to become thinner and may progress to baldness; its texture may become coarse and the colour may become grey or white. Seborrhoeic or 'senile' warts, haemangiomas and other blemishes on the skin are common. Spontaneous rupture of small subcutaneous vessels leads to bruising or 'senile purpura', especially on the hands and arms. The eyes lack lustre and there may be difficulty in focussing. The periphery of the visual field may be restricted, leading to visual inattention. The 'arcus senilis', an opaque ring at the outer edge of the iris, is of no significance. Hearing may be impaired, particularly for high-pitched sounds. Speech may be slower and less distinct. The senses of taste and smell may deteriorate.

Mobility will be reduced and movements such as dressing and undressing will be slower. The gait may become stiff and unsteady, with short shuffling steps. Motor inattention will increase the liability to fall, which is also aggravated by failure of coordination and slowed reactions. There may be a coarse trembling or shaking of the head, lower jaw or hands, which is obvious to the onlooker. Poor foot care, giving rise to bunions, corns or deformed toenails, may also decrease mobility.

Mental effects Almost more important than the physical slowing up is the effect of ageing on the mental faculties. There is usually some decline in intelligence, though this is variable and not noticeable in the majority of old people. Thought processes slow down and elderly people must be allowed to take their time; however, they are able to compensate by drawing on previous experience. Learning continues, although it is more difficult and has to be tackled at a slower pace; practical knowledge is more easily acquired than theoretical. The nurse will often experience this when trying to rehabilitate an elderly patient.

Memory for recent events is one of the earliest mental faculties to become impaired; usually one starts by forgetting names, places and dates. Conversely, events long past may be recalled with great vividness and may be detailed over and over again to the same listener. As a result of this inability to adapt to new thoughts and routines, elderly people like to retain familiar objects and will resist change. They are easily disturbed to the point of confusion by changes in environment, routine and close contacts.

Blunting of the emotions may also occur, with the old person showing no pleasure over joyous events and no apparent sorrow over sad events or bereavements. He may lose all interest in what goes on around him and develop instead an obsessive interest in his own bodily functions, especially bowel habits.

Personal characteristics may be retained in an exaggerated form, and the old person may become a caricature of himself, and fail to conceal his true feeling as he did when younger.

There is therefore a relative preservation of one's intelligence and acquired personal skills into old age. Physical and mental deterioration are balanced by gains in wisdom and experience; serenity should follow withdrawal from the stresses and strains of everyday life. The elderly need peace and quiet, often preferring to be left alone, to give them the opportunity of adjusting to the process of growing old and to reorganize their lives to suit a different pace of living.

The Elderly Population

The discipline of geriatric medicine has developed rapidly since the inception of the National Health Service in 1948. Much credit for this is due to the work of the early pioneers, which is described briefly in the next chapter. But the rapidly increasing elderly population in Great Britain would soon have made the problem clear for all to see. By 1980 the population over 65 will approach the 9 million mark—one retired person for every 3 in employment—and the socio-economic implications of this state of affairs are clear to see. The present size of the geriatric problem is well illustrated in Fig. 1 by the high proportion of handicapped or hospital patients who are over 65.

At present the ratio of over-65s to under-65s (Fig. 2) is

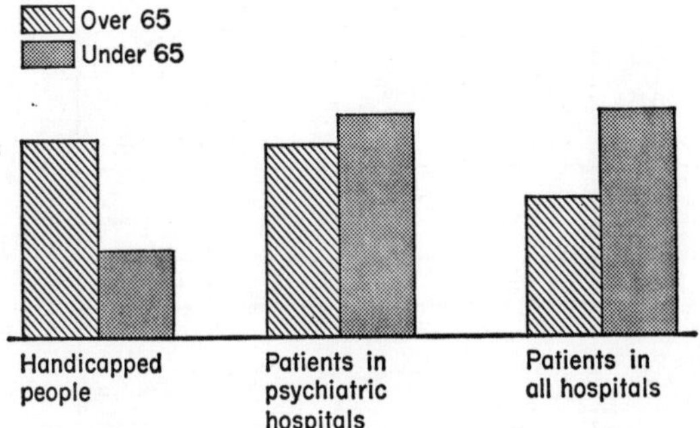

FIG. 1. Hospital patients and handicapped people in Great Britain, over 65 and under 65, as a percentage of the total in each category.

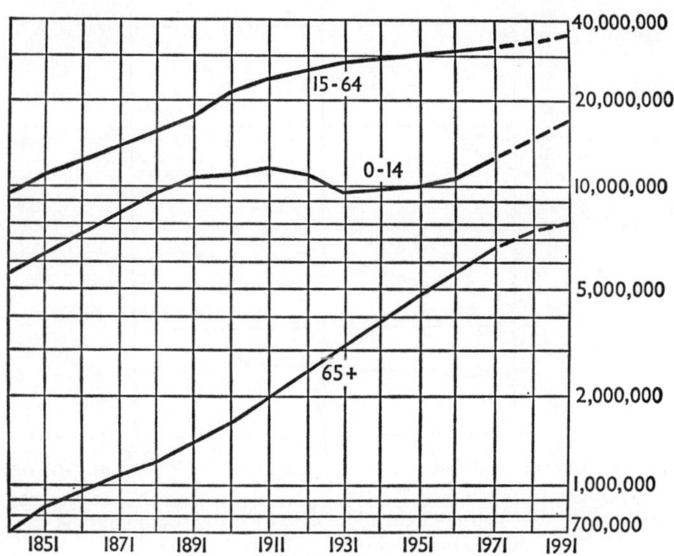

FIG. 2. The proportion of people over 65 in the community at the present time and projected into the future.

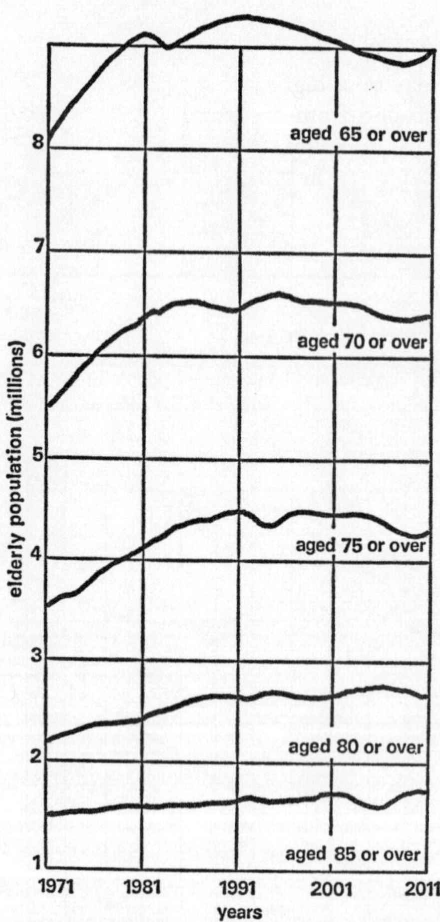

FIG. 3. The distribution of the older elderly in the community, at the present time and projected into the future

about 1:8, but this varies considerably from area to area. On the south coast, for instance, a popular retirement area, the figure may be as high as 1:3.

More alarming from the point of view of the geriatric services is the increasing number of *older* elderly in the community (Fig. 3). In 1900 in Great Britain there were less than half a million people over 75; in 1967 the figure had risen to 2 million, and it is estimated that by 1985 there will be over 3 million. The over-85s will increase by 18% over the next 10 years. The very old, because of their increased vulnerability to all the attendant processes of age, will put added strain on social, geriatric and psychogeriatric services.

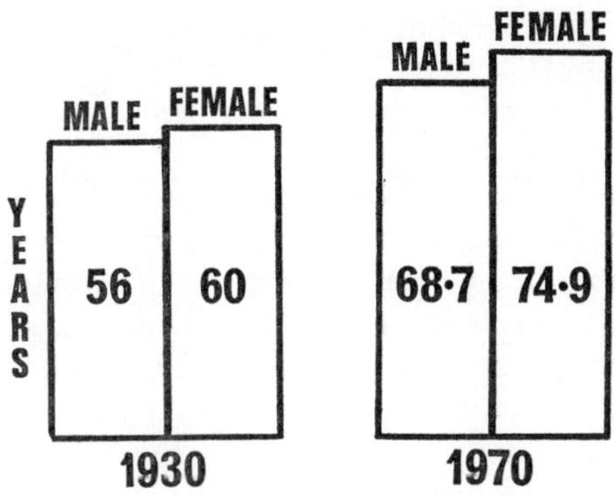

FIG. 4. The expectation of life at birth in 1930 and 1970.

How has this situation arisen? Progress in medicine has mainly benefited children and the middle-aged, particularly by control of infection, advances in surgery and general improvements in infant welfare. Consequently more people are living long enough to experience the degenerative diseases of old age, such as atherosclerosis, arthritis and cancer, where medical science has not advanced so considerably. Despite the overall increase in life span, the expectation of life at 65 has increased by only 1 year in the last 100 years; at 70 it is 10 years and at 80 it is 5 years (Fig. 4).

Social Problems of the Elderly

As many elderly people are among the most deprived members of the community, both financially and socially, the discipline of geriatrics must frequently involve social medicine. In the United Kingdom the single person's retirement pension is about one-quarter of the single person's average earnings and 2·5 million pensioners rely on the supplementary benefit. Old people also tend to live in below-average housing conditions; 1·5 million live alone, 3 in 10 have no inside lavatory, 3 in 10 have no piped hot water. Some 350 000 old people live in a home without a bath, kitchen or inside lavatory.

Conditions for the elderly living in the community vary. Most fortunate are those who have been able to buy their own house during their working lives. However, nearly 100 000 old people live in residential homes, 4000 in special homes for the mentally confused, nearly 37 000 in geriatric units and 52 000 in mental hospitals. Privately owned and rented accommodation so often becomes too large and expensive to maintain when the family have grown up and left home. The houses are often unmodernized and create further problems should the occupant become infirm or disabled. One can see this situation in almost any street of any town or city—the house in need of repair and decoration, the garden running wild due to neglect, the grimy windows and tattered closed curtains.

Elderly people require comfortable, warm, well-lit and convenient accommodation, without steps and stairs. The house should not be isolated, so that help is at hand in an emergency. Specially adapted old people's bungalows or flats (Plate I), warden-controlled flats or 'granny' flats attached as annexes to the houses of younger people are ideal.

TABLE 1. The social problems of the aged sick

Family strain	27%
Relatives cannot cope any longer	
Nearest relative is ill	
Relative cannot stay away from work	
Patient unwanted by family	
Disability disturbing home life	21%
Incontinence or dirty habits	
Completely bed-ridden	
Frequent falls	
Loneliness	15%
Always alone	
Relatives out at work all day	
Mental changes	14%
Confusion	
Nocturnal restlessness	
Wanders and gets lost	
Temperamental or eccentric	
Financial problems	11%
Cannot pay fees of nursing home	
Reluctant landlady	
Other social difficulties	2%
No social problems	10%

After Howell (1970).

Poor housing often leads to loss of independence in the elderly, and at present alternatives are restricted. Breakdown of the extended family unit is common nowadays, and in any case the family is smaller than in the Victorian era, when large families helped to ensure that someone would be available to care for the older members, as they still do in developing countries. In addition, the younger portion of the family tends to move away seeking better employment opportunities, and may even emigrate. Employment of women and earlier marriages have also changed the pattern of the family unit. Domestic help has become an expensive luxury, even for the working woman, and it is difficult to get anyone to 'live in'.

It is not the legal responsibility of the family to care for its elderly, but the moral obligation remains, despite the services provided by the welfare state.

The more one works with the elderly, the more one marvels at the devotion and duty shown by some families to their older members, although households where two, or even three, generations live together, with all their tensions, are becoming less common. It is remarkable how seldom total rejection shows itself, although partial rejection may become apparent in a crisis.

The social problems of the aged sick are summarized in Table 1.

The Geriatric Patient

It is difficult to define the geriatric patient. From a statutory point of view, women qualify for the retirement pension at 60 and men at 65. If we exclude paediatric, mental and obstetric beds, then two-thirds of those which remain are occupied by people in this age group, although it is clear that these are not in the 'geriatric' category other than for chronological reasons. Because of the definitions of old age, there are many combinations and permutations of ageing in each of us; some people remain young in their eighties and others are already old in their fifties or sixties.

For example, an 80-year-old lady, who is entirely independent, but falls and fractures her femur and is subsequently admitted to hospital for surgery, may take a little longer than a younger person to regain mobility and independence before being discharged back to her own home, but she cannot be regarded as a geriatric patient. However, a man aged 55, who is hypertensive and has had a 'stroke', which leaves him partially disabled and dependent on others, possibly with difficulties in communication and with periods of confusion, disorientation and incontinence, may be regarded as a geriatric patient, as he will require the total care approach which will be described later.

Once again it must be stressed that ageing is not a disease, though it may cause some dis-ease. It is a mistake to attribute the troubles of the elderly to senility, implying that nothing can be done about them: apart from anything else, it is disparaging to call anyone senile. The term is invariably used to cover ignorance, and diagnoses such as 'galloping senility' should be avoided.

In old people social, mental and physical handicaps are often present at the same time, and the normal deteriorations of ageing will be present in various degrees: slowing of emotions, poor immediate recall, lessened physical stamina, altered sleep pattern, impaired special senses and impaired adaptation.

The outstanding characteristic of the geriatric, as opposed to other patients, is the occurrence in many cases of multiple pathologies, leading to a number of disabilities. On taking random samples from the elderly in the community an average of 3 disease processes will be found. Each disease alone will not necessarily be lethal, but each will put strain on other diseased organs or tissues. As a result the general health and physical competence of the patient will be impaired, and there will be an eventual breakdown. Should an acute illness be superimposed on this precarious state, then an acute crisis will arise, and the patient will become a geriatric emergency.

An example would be an old person with moderate anaemia, incipient congestive cardiac failure and bronchitis. In this state he might be able to maintain semi-independence; should pneumonia or a urinary infection supervene, however, he will become totally dependent on others. The onset of total dependence often brings to light pre-existing partial dependence.

Another feature of the elderly patient is unreported illness. Whereas the younger patient will report illness himself, the elderly tend to keep their troubles to themselves, adopting the attitude that the illness is due to old age and nothing can be done to help.

A good deal of interest in geriatric medicine lies in the recognition of the boundaries of normal senescence and in the unexpected ways in which diseases are modified in old people. For instance, in the elderly, as in children, the heat-regulating mechanism may be impaired, so an acute infection may not produce the expected rise in temperature or rigor; an old person frequently has bronchopneumonia with a normal or subnormal temperature. In the same way, undue exposure to cold may result in a marked fall in temperature and consequent hypothermia. Sensitivity to pain is reduced and acute appendicitis may occur with little more than discomfort, or a fracture of the femur may be quite painless and go undetected.

Coronary thrombosis leading to myocardial infarction will present with the classical pain in 20% of elderly patients. The usual modes of presentation in the remainder are giddiness, acute confusion, cerebral thrombosis, sudden shortness of breath, increased congestive failure or syncope.

Physical illness may provoke mental confusion in the elderly, and 30% of geriatric patients admitted to hospital are in a state of acute confusion which will subside when the physical conditions have been successfully treated.

Nursing the Geriatric Patient

The elderly patient requires a great deal of understanding, kindness and patience, and no aspect of nursing care makes greater demands on the nurse's qualities of humanity, adaptability, temperament and sheer physical strength. Emphasis must be placed less on cure than on improvement to a level where the patient can become independent again and be accepted back into society. The geriatric unit is therefore not concerned solely with the patient's immediate medical, mental and social problems, but with his functional levels, his reactions to illness and the reaction of the family to him, as well as with economic and social problems. The 'total care approach' demands continuity at all levels of care at home, in hospital and after discharge from hospital.

There are many aspects to the problems of the elderly which the nurse should always bear in mind, for she can do much to maintain the patients' self-respect and dignity.

In old age there is frequently a loss of personal pride, particularly regarding cleanliness and appearance; there is reluctance to change and wash clothing and attend to personal hygiene, probably owing to the effort involved and the lack of any incentive. Feeding habits may deteriorate, becoming messy and neglectful. The nurse must do all she can to counteract these tendencies, although this will not be easy. Many old people become quite out of touch with reality, particularly as it concerns their own disabilities and shortcomings. As a result they will totally reject any help or advice. This trait becomes particularly evident when it is obvious to all but the patient that he cannot continue to live alone and independently. Irritability will take the form of finding fault with everything and everyone. Old people with communication problems often find it difficult to understand what is happening around them; the resulting insecurity will make them possessive of people or property.

The elderly person must be treated as an individual, with a personality of his own, otherwise he will lose his identity and all incentive to go on living. He should be treated like a human being, and not as a mere object which is old, useless and unwanted. To have a feeling of belonging is one of the basic needs, in addition to that for love and affection, which we all share.

The fears of old age are of loneliness and unwantedness and of becoming a burden to one's family. It is important to minimize infirmity when dealing with the old, and this is best achieved by encouraging them to do as much as they can for themselves, no matter how difficult or time-consuming. All these points will go a long way towards maintaining the elderly person's pride, independence and self-respect. It is advantageous not to have too strict a discipline on the wards, with rigid rules. The patients should have some say in their own activities and should be encouraged to express themselves.

The special senses deteriorate with age and problems of failing sight and hearing can create difficulties for the nurse as well as the patient. Inability to communicate seldom brings much sympathy, and this can be most frustrating for the old person if he feels cut off from society. Failing sight and hearing will make the old person withdrawn and further disinclined to accept help, unless the nurse can make the effort to overcome the initial difficulties. It is important to speak slowly and distinctly without shouting, preferably facing the person one is speaking to. Toleration of shortcomings in communication is most important.

If they are not kept occupied and out of bed during the day, elderly people tend to drop off to sleep, and are then less likely to get a good night's rest.

Only when working with the elderly will the nurse develop an understanding of their all-too-many problems and difficulties. She must adopt a positive attitude of mind which will help her in the management of her patients and reward her labours. She should not forget the basic elements of nursing care. When working in a geriatric unit there is always the danger of developing a biased view of the elderly, but the nurse must remember that she sees only about 5% of the old people in the unit's catchment area, and these are the ones in trouble with ill health or social problems. The other 95% remain in the community and live their lives happily with varying degrees of help from the community of which they form a part.

Psychogeriatric Care

Mental illness is associated with loneliness, deprivation, prolonged physical illness and lack of interest or occupation, and so is especially common among the aged. Elderly people suffer from the same type of mental illnesses as the rest of the population, and can be treated in similar ways, frequently with good results. The nurse should remember that some 30% of geriatric admissions are suffering from confusion which will subside when physical symptoms have been adequately treated.

Of the mentally ill in psychiatric hospitals 45% are over 65, and it is estimated that if present trends continue this figure will have increased to 60% by 1985. This is mainly due to the increasing proportion of the population who are over

65. About 1 in 10 old people are thought to suffer from some degree of brain deterioration, leading to various forms of dementia which are so far incurable. Fortunately the condition is often so mild that the sufferer can continue to live at home or in special accommodation for the elderly mentally infirm; for more severe cases the only answer is a mental hospital or long-term geriatric care.

Although the elderly make up only about 13% of the population at present, they account for 33% of suicides, with a higher proportion of men than of women. This may reflect the fact that the social structure of the western world makes it more difficult for an elderly man to care for himself without help.

Paranoid illnesses and depression are particularly common among those living alone. Single old people without relations are twice as likely to be admitted to hospital or to require residential care as are those with families. Frequently the psychiatric disorder may be the continuation or exaggeration of a personality problem established in earlier life.

Hazards of Drug Therapy in the Elderly

There is always a temptation to treat any disease immediately with drugs, but it is easy to make matters worse rather than better by inappropriate or excessive prescribing. In the elderly, drug activity may be modified by a number of factors, including fluctuations in absorption, distribution, excretion and metabolism of drugs. Difficulties in diagnosis, the commonness of multiple pathology and reduced tolerance to drugs due to age or disease all increase the dangers.

Overdosage is particularly likely to occur if the drug being used remains active in the body until it is excreted by the kidneys, because renal function diminishes with old age, even in the absence of detectable disease. There may be a reduction of 30% in the glomerular filtration rate in apparently healthy people over 65.

Complicated drug schedules should be avoided and the minimum number of drugs should be used with the minimum dosages capable of producing the desired effects. The elderly patient with multiple physical illnesses, and possibly mental depression and social problems in addition, is a likely victim for 'polypharmacy' with all its dangers. Moreover the suicide rate is rising among the elderly, and these are just the people for whom large quantities of drugs may be prescribed.

The nurse can help by asking a patient's relatives to bring in *all* his medications when he is admitted to hospital. Dusty old bottles of all shapes, sizes and contents, and in various states of depletion, will accumulate in drawers, on mantelpieces and on bedside tables in any home. Leftovers should be destroyed without exception to prevent self-medication at a later date or the handing on of medicines to friends and neighbours. A look round the home does not take long and is a useful exercise in preventive medicine, whether it is done by the relatives of the patient, the nurse or the doctor. In addition this will make it easy to ensure that the patient is discharged home with only those drugs he really needs.

It is a help to old people to have their medicine bottles clearly labelled with simple and unambiguous instructions. Chemists' labels are often confusing to those with poor eyesight. The nurse should explain the dosages and their timing to the patient and make certain that he understands; she should write down the details if necessary.

Preventive Geriatrics

Prevention of illness is always better than cure, and assistance in its prevention is provided by medical and social agencies, of which the nurse should be aware. Many varieties of service are available, such as voluntary visiting of old people, old people's clubs, day centres, day hospitals, geriatric advice clinics and special housing arrangements. One thing is certain—when an elderly person is in trouble, the sooner help arrives, the better are the chances of successful treatment.

There should be more education and publicity about the problems of old age and the services available to the elderly, particularly by organizations like Age Concern. Pre-retirement courses and semi-retirement schemes will help the old person adapt smoothly to a new style of life, at the same time remaining mentally and physically active and keeping his dignity and self-respect.

Gerontological research into the natural processes of ageing, and more sophisticated prophylaxis against degenerative processes such as obesity, atherosclerosis and arthritis, will do much to lighten the burdens of old age. The general practitioner and his team of nurses and health visitors should be given more facilities for the screening of vulnerable members of the community, with a view to preventing the occurrence of physical, mental or social crises among the elderly and instituting early treatment where necessary. Health visitors and home nurses are often attached to one or more general practices, although they are employed by the Area Health Authority. Some are based in the general practitioners' premises, while others work from the Area Health Authority clinic. The nurse should ensure that she is familiar with the organization of geriatric services in her area, so that she can give advice where necessary.

If admission to the geriatric unit does become necessary, then it should be as soon as possible; the longer the wait for admission the more difficult will be the assessment of the old person and his treatment and reintegration into the community.

2 The Geriatric Unit

Geriatrics, as a special subject in medicine, is relatively new in Great Britain. Up to 30 years ago, that is at the time of the inception of the National Health Service in 1948, care provided in hospitals for the elderly was mainly custodial. The patients were crowded together in shabby buildings reminiscent of the workhouses described by Dickens, with no prospect of their ever going back into the community.

However in 1935, Dr Marjorie Warren, who was on the staff of the West Middlesex Hospital, Isleworth, was made responsible for several hundred old people in a neighbouring workhouse infirmary which the hospital had taken over. She found grossly overcrowded wards of old people, mostly confined to cots, patients with senile dementia, incontinence, contractures, pressure sores and other complications of prolonged bed rest. Severely disabled people and younger chronic sick who were mentally sound were mixed up with the demented. There was no attempt to sort these people into categories and no attempt at treatment. Everything suggested medical neglect and social squalor.

As a result Dr Warren made proposals to improve the situation and in due course laid the foundations on which modern progressive geriatrics in the United Kingdom has been based. The principle was established that the medical profession, having succeeded in prolonging life, should not remain indifferent when the elderly became sick or infirm. Facilities should be made available for elderly people in general hospitals, thus making it possible for full investigations and treatment. 'The creation of a speciality for geriatrics would stimulate better work and initiate research.'

Sadly, Dr Marjorie Warren met an untimely death abroad, in a car accident, just as she was at the height of her pioneer work.

In the next decade the organization of geriatric care in Britain made great strides. In 1940 the National Old People's Welfare Council was formed; 1948 saw the development of a medical society for the care of the elderly, which later became known as the British Geriatric Society. Lord Amulree was the first President and remained so until quite recently. Many of the other founder members still hold office in the society which now has about 600 members. The society has done much to advance policy and research in its field. Geriatric medicine has become a subject in the undergraduate medical curriculum and the Royal College of Physicians now accepts a programme for the training of consultant physicians in geriatric medicine. The discipline of geriatrics has received academic sanction which has culminated in the creation of 8 professorial chairs in the British Isles.

1969 will be regarded as the year in which geriatric departments, which for so long had been at the back of the queue for buildings, staff and equipment, were brought forward and given some of the tools for their difficult task.

Until quite recently most of the developing geriatric units had to be formed in the old workhouse infirmaries which were segregated from the general hospital. These workhouses were mainly built in the Victorian era and usually consisted of the workhouse proper run by a Master and a separate infirmary run by a Matron. The infirmary wards were long, narrow, dingy and overcrowded. It is not difficult to imagine the stigma which was attached to these places when a great number were taken over by the National Health Service in 1948. The early geriatric physicians had to overcome this attitude and improve the conditions in the wards as far as money and upgrading would allow. The general main difficulty was the segregation of the workhouse infirmary from the general hospital; as a result there were no facilities for the investigation or rehabilitation of patients. Suitable staffing was a problem due to the lowly status accorded to persons employed in workhouse infirmaries and with the chronic sick.

In the last few years beds for assessment and rehabilitation have been opened in general hospitals, often built and designed for this specialized work. Now it is the policy of the Department of Health to include geriatric departments in the new district general hospitals.

The Geriatrician

The geriatrician should not only be a good physician, but his skills should include the ability to teach, to organize and to administer. His first priority must be to tackle the needs of the sick, but a programme of preventive care is very important. He leads a large multi-disciplinary team, as geriatrics depends on team work. He is also closely involved with the general practitioner service and community, also the Local Authority and voluntary services. Accordingly the geriatrician has a teaching rôle in both the hospital and the community services.

To establish a really effective service, a programme of regular training for all those involved in the care of the elderly is essential. Geriatric training is required not only by the undergraduate, but also by doctors after qualification, especially general pracitioners, hospital nursing staff, home nurses, health visitors, social workers, occupational therapists and physiotherapists, as about 95% of our elderly still live at home in the community, and a great number of general hospital beds will be occupied by elderly patients. It has been estimated that, excluding paediatric and obstetric hospital beds, nearly two-thirds of the remainder are occupied by elderly people.

The immediate problem for the geriatrician is management of old and chronic sick patients occupying acute medical, surgical and orthopaedic beds. A geriatric unit cannot ease the situation unless enough geriatric beds are available and adequately staffed.

It is important to stress that the aim of the geriatrician is not merely to prolong life which may already be purposeless and burdensome. He aims to keep the elderly healthy, happy and active while they complete their allotted span of years, whatever that may be for each individual. After all, the elderly have already achieved quantity, what they now need is life of good quality.

The Nursing Team

The nurse has to develop an appropriate attitude of mind when dealing with the elderly patients. Many nurses still consider that the care of geriatric patients is the responsibility of other people in another place. They do not realize that they form a vital part of the geriatric unit team and must initiate the rehabilitation of the patients in their care. They are the only staff who maintain a 24-hour contact with patients in hospital; in other words continuity will be provided by a succession of nurses, possibly working in 3 shifts. Apart from close observation of the patient, in addition to their normal duties, they provide the continuity of remedial, social and diversional aspects of care, in the periods when the paramedical staff (physiotherapists, occupational therapists and others) are not on the wards.

As in other wards the nurse has many technical tasks to

perform, but work in a geriatric ward, perhaps more than in any other, demands considerable 'real nursing' skills; sick and elderly people can often be very difficult, but nevertheless they are in great need of compassion and understanding. The work is hard both mentally and physically, and calls for great patience, cheerfulness and optimism.

There is still to be found the attitude that geriatric wards are less demanding in nursing skills than general wards, and need fewer nurses. Several studies have shown that work on a geriatric ward exceeds in quantity and equals in quality that of a general medical ward. Moreover, because of the high turnover in an admission ward operating under a system of progressive patient care, geriatric nursing exceeds general nursing in variety too.

In an acute geriatric admission ward, if the patients are to receive the care they need without undue strain upon the nursing staff, the allocation of nurses should be greater than in general wards. Taking into account holidays, sickness and study time it is recommended that the approved establishment should be on the basis of 1 nurse to 1·25 patients in acute (assessment and rehabilitation) geriatric wards and 1 nurse to 1·5 patients in long stay wards.

For nurses to develop the right attitude towards the elderly patient and not to regard them as 'chronic sick' or see their problems as due to the irreversible process of ageing, it is essential that they become active members of a multi-disciplinary team.

Special training in this branch must be arranged in order to equip them for this hard and difficult skill in nursing, which is so often rewarding but may at times be disappointing and frustrating. Geriatric nursing is a challenge not to be indulged by the faint-hearted.

The Functions and Organization of the Unit

The functions are:

1. To maintain the functional independence—physical, mental and social—of the aged person and so postpone or avoid institutional treatment.
2. To teach.
3. To undertake research.

First, it is essential to have an adequate number of beds for the elderly population in the unit catchment area. The normal yard-stick is 10 beds per 1000 but this, of course, will vary according to other facilities in the area such as nursing homes, welfare homes and various forms of sheltered housing. Because the number of beds is large, possibly several hundred, widely disseminated throughout the area, and because requests for beds are made from many sources, such as community, welfare homes and other hospital departments, it is essential to have a central office with full secretarial staff; this ensures coordination and good communication during working hours.

The office and main unit for acute admissions should be sited within a general hospital. This enables the patients to be investigated satisfactorily with facilities for laboratory and radiological investigations. The opinions of consultants in other specialties are more easily obtained.

In-patients

As will be seen in Fig. 5 wards are allocated for special functions. It has been shown by experience that a system of progressive patient care provides the most effective results. The main criticism of this form of care is the sometimes frequent moves for patients, depending on their progress or deterioration. All patients are admitted initially to the *acute assessment and intensive care wards*. In these wards they will be thoroughly examined clinically, mentally and functionally. Routine investigations and any other investigations indicated will be carried out. After a period of 4–6 weeks' treatment a decision will be taken regarding the patient's future. It has been found that approximately a third of the patients will die during this initial period, a third will recover sufficiently to be discharged back to the community, possibly with more support or supervision than they were receiving prior to admission. The remaining third can be transferred to a *rehabilitation continued nursing care ward*, where the emphasis will be upon regaining personal independence—the ability to wash, visit the lavatory, dress and walk. During this phase of rehabilitation further treatment and nursing will be required. Alternatively, the patient will be moved to a long-stay annexe if he is unable to cope with the rehabilitation programme. This is to be regarded as a last resort.

When a patient recovers reasonable independence but for various social reasons is unable to return to the community he will be moved to an *ambulant ward* or '*halfway house*' with a low staff/patient ratio. Ideally a self-care unit or flat should be attached to this ward. Patients may then live independently but under supervision until the social workers have made arrangements for suitable accommodation in the community. This part of the unit is especially useful for patients returning home to live alone.

Some patients cannot respond to treatment or rehabilitation and they may need so much nursing care that they are unable to return to the community under any circumstances. These patients are moved to one of the *long-stay* annexes when a bed is available (see Chapter 9).

Specialized wards In some well established units there will be wards run jointly with other specialties.

Psychogeriatric assessment wards These are wards where elderly patients will be seen by the geriatrician, psychiatrist and, if necessary, social worker of the social services department. After a suitable assessment the patient will be transferred either to a geriatric unit ward or to a psychiatric ward for further treatment and care. This arrangement lessens the likelihood of the patient being misplaced and receiving the wrong care, which is to his detriment. Both the acute geriatric and psychiatric beds will be situated in the new district general hospitals, thus obviating the need for psychogeriatric assessment wards as liaison and communication between the two will be greatly improved.

An orthopaedic/geriatric unit This has been shown to improve the outcome of patients, particularly those with fractured femurs, amputations and following mobilization surgery. The surgery and postoperative care is supervised by the orthopaedic surgeon and his staff, whereas the general care of the patient and his rehabilitation is the responsibility of the geriatric unit. Joint ward rounds are carried out by both consultants.

A hemiplegic unit orientated to intensive rehabilitation of 'stroke' patients increases the patient's prospects of maximum recovery.

Out-patient Care

The increasing load of hospital care is being carried more and more on an out-patient basis. The out-patients department is for those who need hospital treatment, and have been referred by their general practitioner, but whose case does not warrant admission on an in-patient basis. The out-patients department also follows up patients after discharge (see Chapter 12). Remember that this may be the patient's first introduction to hospital, and first impressions are important. If the patient is rushed in, has a hasty conference with the doctor, and is rushed out again without understanding the plans proposed or the reasons for the investigation, it will not be surprising if he cannot be persuaded to attend a second time. A leisurely clinic in the unit is more efficacious for the elderly and will encourage the patients to attend and the practitioners to refer their patients. New patients are seen and frequently dealt with on an out-patient basis using all the facilities and expertise of the unit and good community service liaison. A well run out-patient department will play an important part in the preventive programme.

Relatives are also encouraged to attend for advice and to help the elderly patient as necessary. *Relatives' clinics* are also useful for all concerned especially when there are social problems and difficulty in management at home.

Because geriatric out-patients are time-consuming, only a very few patients can be seen at the clinic and they mostly have to be brought by ambulance. Follow-up clinics after a patient is discharged from the wards or Day Hospital will enable the unit to keep a watchful eye on the patient until final discharge.

Treatment in a day hospital is another type of out-patient care, but it occupies such a central place in the geriatric unit that a special section is given to it (pp. 33–38).

Domiciliary Visits

When a crisis arises in the patient's home the consultant physician in geriatrics may visit the patient at the request of his general practitioner. It is very useful to see the patient in his domestic background. Following a history and a full clinical examination including assessment of functional ability and activities of daily living, the relatives and those involved in support (so often a kindly neighbour) may be interviewed. The suitability of the accommodation may be assessed and, if possible, the financial status. It can be helpful for the home nurse, health visitor or social worker also to attend. The geriatrician is then able to get a much clearer picture of the problem and therefore assess the degree of recovery and rehabilitation required for the patient to continue to live in the existing environment.

Following the visit the patient may be treated at home, admitted to the geriatric unit, recommended for day hospital attendance or given more community support with possibly a recommendation for residential accommodation. The social worker from the geriatric unit may then be asked to visit the house to deal with any social problems. She will liaise with the health visitor from the primary care team or social worker from the Social Services department.

The health visitor is a highly qualified trained nurse who has also been trained in social medicine; she is the ideal person to carry all aspects of preventive medicine and nursing into the community. The health visitor is often attached to family doctors in group practices. She is able to give help and advice to the elderly on diet, cooking, home safety and matters of hygiene. At the same time she is able to advise on statutory or supplementary benefits and which departments will supply various aids. It is not part of her function to carry out any practical nursing procedures.

In some areas the Health District will second a health visitor to the geriatric unit. This specialist health visitor sees the patients when they are in hospital and then follows them up when they return home, thereby ensuring any recommended treatment is continued at home, and will assess that the patient is managing within the limits of disability (see also Chapter II).

Holiday Beds

Most geriatric units run a system of holiday beds throughout the year. These beds are not to give the patients a holiday, but to give the hard-pressed relatives a rest and the chance of a holiday. Special beds may be set aside for the purpose and the patient returns home at the end of the prescribed period. While he is in hospital, an assessment and any investigations indicated are carried out. It is good for the staff in the unit to see and to marvel at just what some relatives have to cope with at home, year in and year out, often in extremely difficult conditions. Again, the relatives are more inclined to continue their arduous task if they can look forward to an occasional break. Those patients just requiring supervision are accepted on the same basis by local authority homes during the summer in some areas.

In–Out Scheme

The unit may share the care of a long-stay patient with the relatives, on a 6-weeks-in and 6-weeks-out basis. In this way two patients will use the same bed alternately, this relief will often enable relatives to keep a difficult nursing problem in the community for much longer.

Five-day Wards

This form of care is increasing in popularity. Selected patients are admitted on Monday and discharged home on Friday evening. It has been shown that the sharing of care does not prejudice the improvement of suitable patients. This type of ward is much easier to staff, although the proportion of trained staff requires to be higher. The accent is on rehabilitation and patients receive treatment for several weeks but for a limited period only.

Visiting

Visiting is usually open from 9 a.m. to 9 p.m. Relatives and friends, who are themselves often elderly, are encouraged to visit as frequently as possible. It is beneficial for the patients to see people from the community coming and going. The ward sister often encourages the visitors to carry out small tasks such as feeding, giving drinks or reading to the patient.

The Unit and the Hospital

Fig. 5 illustrates a geriatric unit with the office in the middle as the nerve centre for administration. Round this are the categories of in-patient care, out-patient care, special wards and general hospital services.

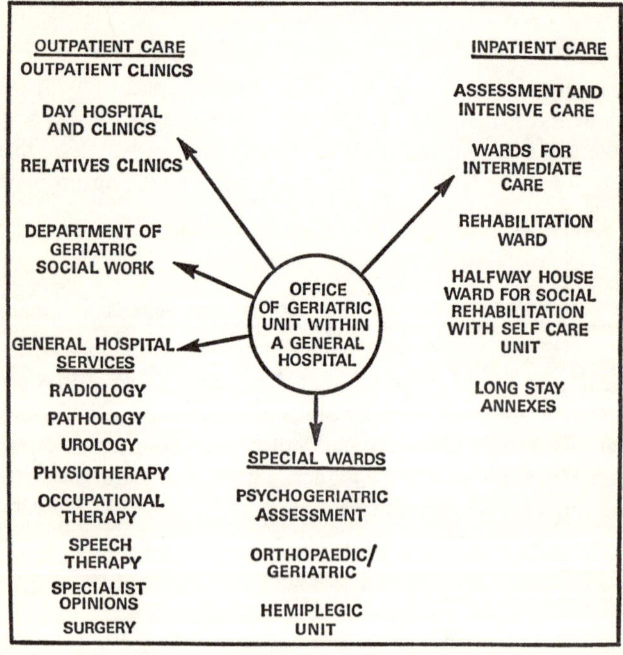

FIG. 5. The geriatric unit and the hospital.

The Unit and the Community

In Fig. 6 the geriatric unit has been placed in two larger circles to represent the community. The total now represents the district geriatric services. One can immediately see how involved are the many facets of care and help for the elderly.

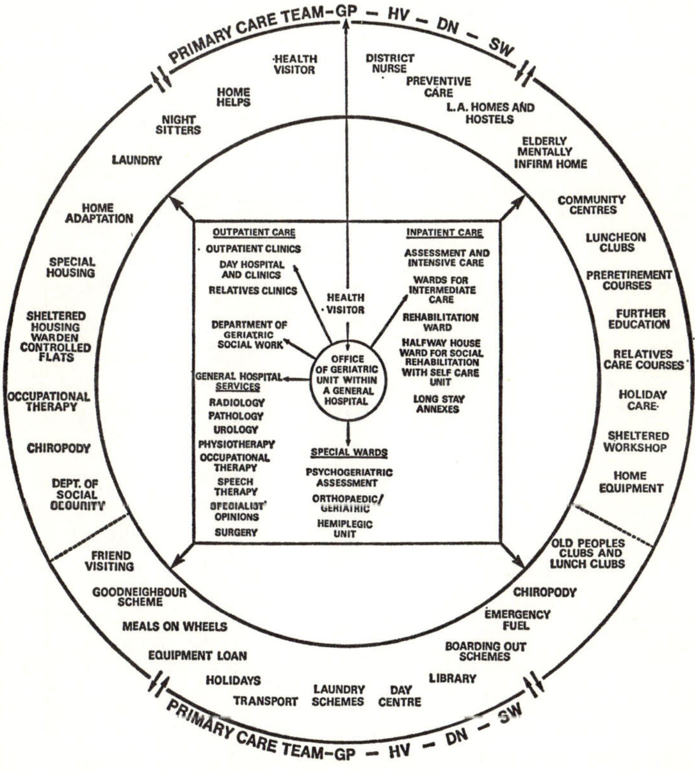

FIG. 6. District geriatric services.

The upper part of the circle shows the numerous services provided by the social services department and other statutory bodies. The lower part of the circle shows some of the facilities provided by the voluntary services. The general practitioner is shown on the periphery of the diagram and it can be seen that he and his team, being in the front line, have access to the geriatric unit facilities, the statutory and voluntary services.

Case Conferences

It has been said previously that geriatrics is essentially team work, due to the multi-disciplinary expertise involved in the management of a patient, both whilst he is in the unit and when he returns to the community. For the structure illustrated to function properly to the patient's advantage, there must be good communication and liaison between doctors, nurses, therapists and social workers. Unit case conferences are therefore often held either before or after ward rounds. Longer case conferences which include representatives of the area social services department, will be called frequently to consider, for example, the environment to which the patient will be discharged and the facilities available. The conference will discuss progress, rehabilitation programme, social problems and arrangements for the patient's discharge from hospital. It is important to consider the problems after discharge before the medical conditions have been treated and the rehabilitation programme completed, so that when the time comes to return the patient to the community there is no delay for domestic reasons. Disappointment and delay leads to deterioration in patients who have reached their maximum ability, following all the efforts made both on their part and that of others.

Day Care

The Day Hospital The geriatric day hospital is a building to which patients may come or be brought in the morning and where they spend several hours in therapeutic activity, returning home the same day. As most of the patients will have to be brought by motor transport, good access is essential.

The day hospital is open daily for 5 days a week and patients may attend as frequently as is necessary, although the majority come on 1 or 2 days only. There is normally accommodation for 20 to 50 patients per day.

The day hospital in a geriatric unit has a marked effect on the morale of the unit, both staff and patients alike, but for it to function efficiently it is essential that there should be complementary day establishments within the geriatric service. These include day centres, day clubs, workshops for the elderly and local authority day care.

The Department of Health has estimated that 2 day hospital places are necessary for every 1000 of the population over 65. It has been shown that, with proper day care facilities, full-time admission to hospital could be avoided in about 1 out of 12 patients. One in 20 would have admission delayed and an earlier discharge from hospital would be possible in about 1 in 10 cases.

The majority of geriatric units have the advantage of a day hospital within the unit, and many of those who do not, have plans to erect one in the next few years. Some are found within the geriatric hospital, some in the general hospital and some are entirely separate. It is usually the central point of the hospital's medical and social services and the heart of the geriatric unit. Some are run by an occupational therapist, some by a state-registered nurse, and some jointly, but in nearly all cases a qualified nurse and therapist are in attendance.

Geriatric day hospitals began in the 1950s when out-patients attended wards or out-patient departments for the day only. It is interesting to note that several psychiatric day hospitals developed in the previous decade. The first purpose-built geriatric day hospital in this country was at Oxford in 1958, but numbers have grown rapidly since then and there were 119 by 1970.

Functions and benefits of the day hospital. The day hospital is a *therapeutic* unit. Its functions are:

1. Functional assessment.
2. Medical investigation.
3. Maintenance to prevent deterioration.
4. Short-term rehabilitation.
5. Long-term rehabilitation.
6. Support for relatives.

Its particular benefits, in relation to other forms of care and treatment, are:

1. Treatment for former in-patients can continue in a new environment which raises interest and morale.
2. A midway stage between hospital and home helps the patient adjust psychologically to discharge.
3. In-patients and out-patients can mix, which provides social contact.
4. Hospital beds are saved and nurses are released as staffing is required 5 days a week only.
5. The burden on relatives is relieved without removing responsibility.

By far the most important service provided by these units are those of physical rehabilitation and medical supervision.

Next in order of priority is maintenance therapy for those who are particularly frail. The third requirement concerns patients needing social care who are too frail to be looked after elsewhere.

Other services available in most day hospitals are dentistry, chiropody and audiometric services (hearing aids). Ophthalmic opinion in the general hospital will also be accessible on an out-patient basis.

The geriatric social worker will interview patients and relatives on matters regarding the social services, finance and allowances. She will also advise on all statutory and voluntary services.

Attached to the day hospital, either separately or in combination, there will be a technical workshop with a technical instructor in charge. Patients participate in occupations making various aids and articles requiring special movements as part of their rehabilitation.

The majority of patients suffer from a major disability such as locomotor disease, a stroke or various forms of arthritis, but commonly they will have multiple conditions. On first day attendance the patient is assessed, first by clinical examination, then for any medical investigations and treatment required, then for other forms of therapy such as physiotherapy, occupational therapy and speech therapy.

When a patient has reached the stage of maximum benefit resulting in a plateau of functional ability then consideration must be given to discharge, at either a review clinic or a case conference. Some patients will require further support; they may be introduced to a club or day centre. It is important to hold regular clinics for initial assessment, arranging a programme of therapy, review of progress and final discharge. In this way one can ensure a regular flow of patients through the day hospital, thus creating places for new patients. It has been shown that rehabilitation patients attend for periods of about three months. On the other hand, social patients may attend for a year or more and both they and their relatives become very easily dependent on the day hospital. Social intercourse is obviously valuable, particularly for the many patients who live isolated at home, but this should not be the only reason for the patient occupying a place in the day hospital. Attendance at a day centre may be just as helpful.

Fig. 7 illustrates where the admissions come from and to where they are eventually discharged.

The patient's day. Before the patient attends the day hospital, he and his relatives will have had clear instructions as to the days he is required to attend, so that he is ready when the ambulance man calls in the morning. The ambulance man can report a patient's difficulty in attending so that this can be quickly investigated by the social worker, health visitor or general practitioner.

The patients arrive in sitting ambulances which may have been collecting several people from a particular area. The ambulance crews are specially picked for their patience and understanding attitude to elderly people, as not infrequently the patient is not ready or is even still in bed. Incidentally, the ambulance service is the most costly single item in day hospital care.

On arrival the patients are greeted by the staff and given refreshments. The morning is spent on individual therapy, clinics, clinical examination and medical treatment. Assessments are carried out on activities of daily living—dressing, the ability to manage lavatory facilities, bathing, self-care, kitchen. Throughout the day baths, chiropody and hairdressing continue. A launderette is usually available so that patients can get their washing done while visiting the hospital.

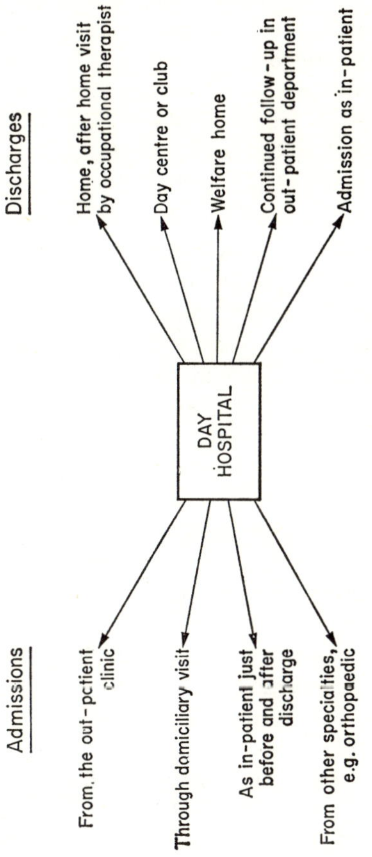

FIG. 7. The day hospital.

After lunch, which is a social occasion as well as ensuring satisfactory nutrition, the patients will have a rest. The afternoon is spent on music and group movement, art, entertainment and crafts. Sometimes a church service will be arranged. At the end of the afternoon, following tea, the ambulance will call to take the patients home.

Usually there is a library trolley with special large print books available. The Women's Royal Voluntary Service trolley shop comes round with toiletries, confectionery and other articles and is a great source of pleasure to many patients who are often unable to get to the shops.

Relatives are encouraged to attend the day hospital at least once to discuss any problems arising at home and to see what the elderly patient is able to do and how to encourage activity at home. If necessary the therapist and social worker will make a home visit to assess special aids and adaptations necessary for the patient to gain as much independence as possible in the community.

Day Centres It is important to differentiate between day hospitals and day centres. The latter provide social facilities only and are run by voluntary lay workers with a nurse in attendance; no specialist medical services are provided and they are not normally attached to hospitals. However the elderly person can attend as frequently and as long as he wishes. Bathing and chiropody services are available, and usually also a launderette. Day centres, like day hospitals, provide social contact and distraction for the lonely and housebound. They are suitable for those who require the minimum of medical supervision.

Summary

To summarize, the main function of the geriatric unit is to provide a comprehensive medical service to maintain the elderly in the community. This objective is achieved by:

1. *Diagnosis*
   - *a.* Fully competent medical team
   - *b.* Accommodation for both in- and out-patients
   - *c.* Modern equipment

2. *Rehabilitation*
   - *a.* Staff:
     specially trained nurses
     occupational therapists
     physiotherapists
     speech therapists
     rehabilitation aides
     psychologists
     chiropodists
   - *b.* Accommodation:
     special departments
     day hospital
     day wards
     hemiplegic units
   - *c.* Apparatus

3. *Reintegration*
   - *a.* Case conferences
   - *b.* Relatives' clinics
   - *c.* Health visitors or social workers for assessment of home conditions
   - *d.* Interviews with geriatric social worker
   - *e.* Liaison with social services—home helps, warden controlled flats, welfare organizations
   - *f.* Liaison with home nurses
   - *g.* Liaison with voluntary organizations
   - *h.* Psychiatric social workers
   - *i.* Cooperation of general practitioner and his team

4. *Maintenance*
   a. Follow-up clinics
   b. Home visits by occupational therapist, social worker or health visitor
   c. Day hospital
   d. Day centre
   e. Day clubs

To summarize, to work efficiently the geriatric unit needs an organization of its own, involving admissions, discharges, transfers, domiciliary visiting, after-care arrangements, case conferences and liaison meetings. There must be good co-operation and communication with general practitioners, relatives, other hospitals, social services and voluntary organizations.

It is essential to have good team spirit, with all members of the multi-disciplinary team working towards the common goal, that of ensuring their elderly patients remain in the community whilst they live their allotted span, happily, healthily and actively.

3 General Nursing Care of the Elderly Patient

Admission to Hospital

Admission of the elderly patient to hospital is never a very welcome procedure, and the nurse should help to make it as easy and as pleasant as possible. It has often been preceded by a visit by the consultant geriatrician to the patient's home; he will have explained to both the patient and the relatives the reasons for admission and the environment into which the patient will go. The patient is generally acutely ill and requires hospitalization for treatment of this acute illness. Very often the acute illness is superimposed upon a chronic disability. The crisis leading to complete dependency often brings to light an unsuspected semi-dependent state.

One patient admitted to the unit had recently suffered a cerebrovascular accident leaving her with a left hemiplegia. She had been treated during the past years for rheumatoid arthritis, diabetes mellitus, ischaemic heart disease and hypertension; she had come to terms with all these disabilities and was leading a full and independent life, living alone in a bungalow. However, after her cerebrovascular accident she required a period of hospitalization in order to benefit from all the rehabilitation services, and to learn to live with yet another disability.

Sometimes the chronic disease has progressed to such a degree that the patient can no longer manage at home. The geriatric unit investigates and treats the patient, then aims towards rehabilitation so that he is fit to return home, where he can live a fuller and more independent life. Whatever support and aids he may need can be organized while he is in hospital.

Occasionally the patient does not respond to treatment as anticipated, or the illness has progressed so that he is unable to respond and may require permanent hospitalization. Holiday beds are available in most units to give relatives a chance to rest and perhaps take a holiday. Some units arrange intermittent admissions to help the relatives cope with severe disability.

Loss of independence, a change of surroundings and confrontation by innumerable strange faces often precipitates a temporary degree of confusion and even resentment within the patient. Reception of the patient on arrival is most important in helping to create the right atmosphere from the beginning, a cheerful welcome from the staff, after which he is shown quietly to his own locker and bed, and given a cup of tea or coffee. The welcome extended has a great bearing on the patient's ability to settle into the ward routine and will also have a beneficial effect on the cooperation received from the relatives. All these things help to allay the patient's fear. He should also be shown the layout of the ward and the toilet facilities available.

The nurses' approach to the patient is important. The patient should be addressed by his correct name and not by some term of endearment. The name should always be clearly written above the bed for all to see. When addressing the patient the nurse should face the patient and talk to him at his level, so that he can see the nurse's expression and lip movement, as can be seen in Plate IV; the nurse must not stand over him, addressing him above or behind his head.

One lady aged 98 years, admitted from an old people's home, was quite amazed to find she had come into hospital when she saw all the empty beds, as she had no idea that patients were not confined to their beds while receiving treatment!

When the nurse has seen the patient comfortably installed, and introduced him to the patient in the next bed, his suitcase is unpacked and all his belongings placed in his locker. At the same time the nurse can see if he has any valuable articles with him. Many elderly people bring all their worldly goods with them, including large sums of money and valuable jewellery. With the patient's consent these should be either sent home with the relatives, or locked away in the hospital safe. The hospital authorities are not responsible for the patient's property. If he insists on keeping it, this should be made clear to him at the time.

Relatives

Relatives often accompany the patient into hospital and they too should be given a warm and friendly welcome. Their help and cooperation will be needed during the patient's stay, and therefore their reception is of great importance. They are often upset at their mother or father being admitted to a geriatric unit rather than the medical ward, and if the nurse explains the work of the unit at the beginning, resentment and fears can be allayed.

Accurate information can be obtained from the relatives as to the patient's age, address, family doctor and other particulars. Ideally the unit should arrange open visiting hours, so that relatives and friends can come and go at their own convenience. The nurse should try to encourage the relatives to visit at hours when they can help with some of the patient's care, such as feeding, bathing or walking.

Often relatives are frightened by the hospital atmosphere and the bustle of the staff, and no longer feel competent to do what they have been doing so admirably at home. Some also feel they have done enough and are relieved to sit back and have a rest. One devoted daughter, who had looked after a rather trying mother and was really in need of a rest, insisted on visiting twelve hours a day and greatly impeded her mother's progress, despite tactful remarks from the nursing staff, social workers and the general practitioner.

Routine Observations

On admission patients should be weighed routinely and subsequently weekly during their stay in hospital, as weight gains and losses are important and have a direct bearing on their diagnosis and future treatment.

On admission urine should be tested for acidity, specific gravity, sugar, acetone, albumen, blood and bile. The use of Bili-labstix makes all this a quick and simple procedure. Many early diabetics, who have remained undiagnosed until admission, have been detected in this way. A clean specimen of urine should be sent to the laboratory for analysis, as urinary tract infections are common in old age.

It is usual to observe the patient's temperature, pulse and respiration for one week following admission; if all is normal during this time the procedure is then discontinued and only recommenced when necessary. Blood pressure is also recorded for one week, so that a clear pattern of blood pressure can be evolved. It must be remembered that patients suffering from giddiness and falls should have their blood pressure recorded both lying and standing in order to eliminate postural hypotension.

Daily recording of bowel function is important and aperients should be administered in the evening as necessary. Use of the patient's regular aperient may often allay anxiety over precipitant bowel action, but Dorbanex suspension and Senokot have proved to have a gentle and efficient action. Administration of glycerine or Dulcolax suppositories may relieve discomfort following absence of bowel action for 2 or 3 days, but an enema saponis is usually no more uncomfortable and has a more efficient action.

General Nursing Care

The nurse must consider the general care of the patient confined to bed.

Blanket Bath

A daily blanket bath is essential where the patient is unable to bathe in the bathroom and usually much appreciated. The nurse must tell the patient of her intention to carry out the procedure, close the window and offer the patient a commode or bedpan. The nurse will then lay her trolley which will contain:

Clean bed linen and night clothes if necessary
Washing bowl
Patient's own soap, two flannels, two towels
Patient's brush and comb
Mouth tray or mouth-wash and dish
Jug and bucket if a basin is not near at hand.

If the patient is able, he should be encouraged to help as much as possible with the procedure. The bed is stripped, leaving the patient covered by a bath blanket and another blanket if it is a cold day. The face is washed first. Then, starting with each arm, a small area of the body at a time is exposed, washed and dried, the rest being kept covered and warm. The nurse must make sure the water is really hot, so that the patient does not receive a tepid wash. Streaming the patient's hands and feet is very refreshing. The hand or foot is held over the bowl and warm water is trickled over it between the fingers or toes. The water is changed before washing the patient's back, when he should be turned on alternate sides as necessary.

Having completed the washing, the patient will be re-dressed and the bed remade. Attention will then be paid to the hair, nails and mouth. Before leaving the patient, the nurse should ensure that a drink, glasses, handbag or wallet and book are all near at hand.

Position in Bed

The patient's position in bed is important, as so often the elderly find it difficult to be comfortable. Arranging the right number of pillows so that the patient can sit without sliding down the bed, and if necessary enjoy a meal there, is an art. The well-used 'armchair' with 5 pillows is normally the most effective, as demonstrated in Fig. 8.

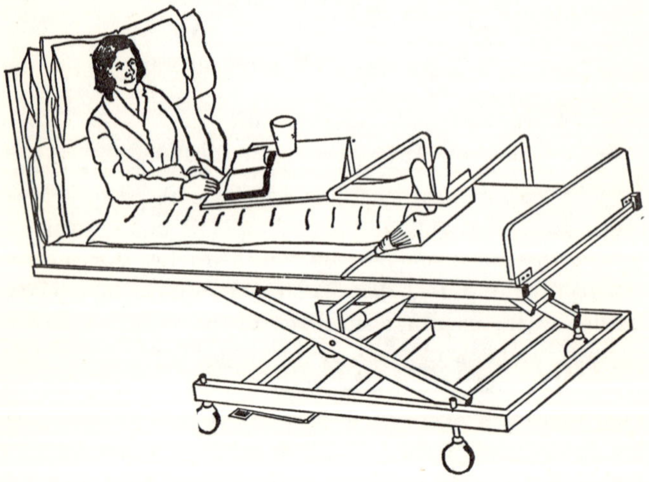

FIG. 8. The correct position for an elderly patient in bed.

A bed cradle should always be used for the following reasons:

1. To allow the elderly patient to move his legs without being impeded by heavy bedclothes.
2. To prevent pressure on the heels.
3. In the case of the hemiplegic patient, to prevent foot drop with the aid of a pillow and board.

When a bed cradle is used, a soft light blanket or bed socks are often much appreciated. Care should be taken in positioning the cradle and seeing that it is high enough above the mattress. It has been known for a patient with very frail skin as the result of prolonged steroid therapy, to knock his legs against the cradle, and as a result in one case to require 10 stitches in his legs.

Cot sides should only be erected for the helpless patient to prevent him falling out of bed; the hemiplegic may be in need of support on the affected side (Fig. 9). In cases of confusion, raised cot sides tend to increase the difficulties, and injuries will be more severe if the patient climbs over the top. In these cases it is far better to nurse the patient with the mattress on the floor.

Pressure Areas

Pressure areas should be treated 2–4-hourly, depending on the condition and mobility of the patient, and his position changed. This subject is discussed in more detail in Chapter 6.

Oral Hygiene

Oral toilet is also necessary and should be performed 2–4-hourly, again depending on the patient's condition. A tray for this purpose, as shown in Plate V, should be re-set twice daily and not left by the bedside to accumulate dust.

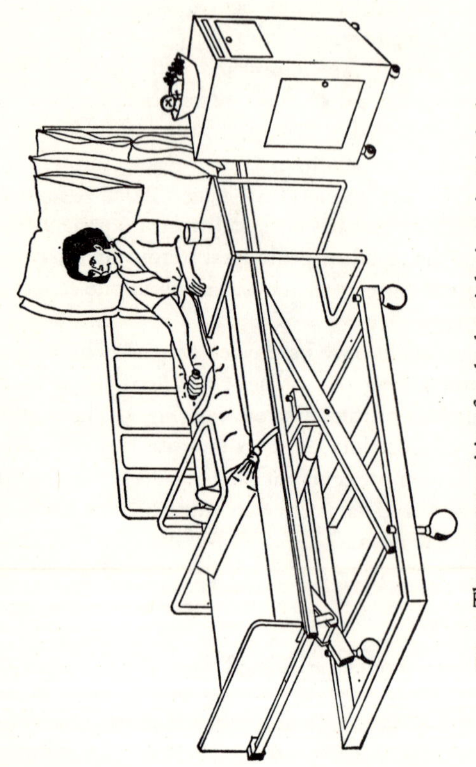

FIG. 9. The correct position for the hemiplegic patient in bed.

The most effective method of cleaning the mouth of the patient who is unable to help himself, is by using a disposable glove, with a piece of gauze wrapped round the finger and dipped in a solution of thymol compound. Artery forceps wrapped with gauze may also be used. Orange sticks must not be used for this purpose as they are dangerous and can penetrate the gums.

A very dirty mouth may benefit from being cleaned with a solution of one part hydrogen peroxide to three parts warm water. *Monilia* infection occurring in the mouth must be treated with a course of nystatin or amphotericin. Finally the mouth can be swabbed with glycerine to encourage salivary secretion. Dry lips can be moistened with petroleum jelly. The nurse must be aware of drugs and food particles collecting in the corners of the mouth; these can lead to ulceration and infection. When this is liable to occur, the mouth should be well cleaned after every meal. It is also important to encourage frequent drinks, as the elderly are loath to take fluids even when they are able and a drink is available.

Lifting

Much of the nurse's time within the geriatric unit is spent lifting, and it is essential that she is taught to do this correctly so that she does not suffer any injury to herself. Elderly people and especially hemiplegic patients are not always able to cooperate fully owing to their disabilities and therefore orthodox lifts are not always used.

The easiest method of lifting a patient up in bed, is for the nurse to place one arm under the patient's arm and grasp her wrist, and the other arm under the patient's thigh and grasp the wrist of the second nurse (Fig. 10).

In order to lift the patient into a chair from the bed, it is

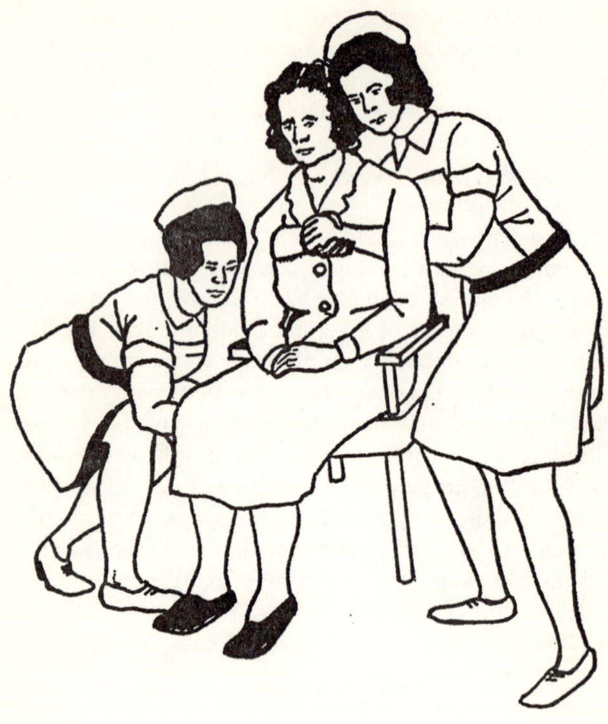

FIG. 10A. Correct method of lifting an elderly patient from a chair.

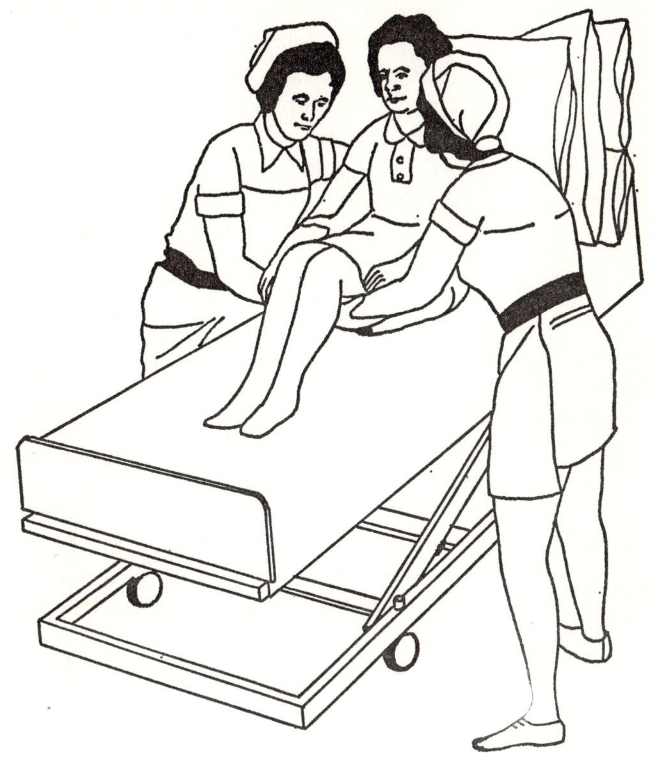

FIG. 10B. Correct method of lifting an elderly patient into bed

often easier for one nurse to be behind the patient, placing her arms across the patient's chest, and for the second nurse to face the patient and lift the patient from the thighs. It is important for the nurse to remember to lift the patient well clear of the bed, and not to drag her up the bed causing friction sores. There must always be 2 nurses to lift, and the nurse must remember to bend her knees, not her back.

Clothing

Patients feel more at home wearing their own clothes wherever possible, and once they are over their acute illness they are encouraged to be up and dressed. Particular importance is laid upon shoes, which should provide good support and comfort. If possible shoes rather than slippers should be worn, although it is often quite a battle to convert some patients to wear shoes after years of only ever wearing slippers. An arrangement with the local shoe shop is often helpful when fitting the patient with new shoes. All clothes and shoes should be marked on arrival as it is amazing how quickly articles (especially underwear) disappear.

Care of Hair

A geriatric unit should view the patient as a whole and not just consider his acute illness. Thus a visit to the unit is a good time to remedy some of the smaller problems also. A haircut and shampoo are often appreciated by those living alone and quite frequently cases of seborrhoea can be treated with medicated shampoos such as Sebbix and severe cases with selenium disulphide. It is usually unnecessary to wash the hair in bed, and this can be done in the bath or shower room. Most units have a hairdresser who visits weekly, and the renewal of a permanent wave or set will often do much to boost the patient's morale.

Deafness and Hearing Aids

Difficulty in hearing has often been accepted as a hazard of old age for which there is no remedy, although in many cases the ears are filled with wax and benefit from being syringed. Olive oil drops for two days before treatment are a help when syringing is needed or a wax softener, such as Cerumol, can be used.

Some patients may need a hearing aid and can be referred to the ear, nose and throat department while in hospital. Those who already have an aid often need assistance as well. Some may have difficulty penetrating the wax. One elderly nun was convinced her aid was no good, yet when she removed the ear-piece it was completely blocked with wax. Even porridge has been discovered there!

While the patient is in hospital it is often a good time for the hearing aid to be overhauled by the audiometrician. Broken parts can be replaced and new batteries can be supplied. New ear moulds can be taken if needed and new pieces fitted. Batteries should be changed every 2 weeks and a good supply should be readily available. The irritating whistle of hearing aids is caused by the amplifier being too near the receiver, and this can be easily remedied.

One must remember that a hearing aid does not improve intelligibility of speech and one must still speak clearly and slowly. If the patient has just acquired a new aid, great patience must be exercised and encouragement given to him to use it. Initial use is very tiring and should only be for short periods of time in a quiet place, as background noises are also amplified and can be very distressing.

Sight and Spectacles

Spectacles may need to be checked and a visit to the optician can usually be arranged. These also should be inconspicuously identified with the patient's name on admission, as they can be easily mislaid and not every owner can recognize his own glasses. The ophthalmologist is always available to see patients with abnormalities of vision and advise them what needs to be done.

Teeth

Decaying teeth are often seen and referred to the dentist if necessary. Ill-fitting dentures may also be remedied while in hospital. These too should be identified with a denture maker to prevent loss. Patients often arrive without their dentures, which they have not worn for years, due to a fault or discomfort. Some small faults may be easily corrected if they are brought into hospital.

Teeth, false or natural, should be cleaned every evening. If the patient is unable to do this for himself, the nurse should do so, soaking them as necessary in a specific denture cleaner. Many elderly people prefer not to be seen without false teeth and usually replace them for the night, after cleaning.

Nails

Nails benefit from a manicure, especially toenails which may have been totally neglected. A visiting chiropodist is an asset to treat onychogryphosis (over-grown, horny toenails), hallux valgus (bunions) and corns, all of which result in the patient wearing ill-fitting footwear and find difficulty in walking.

Mrs X., a retired nurse aged 81 years, was referred to the geriatrician with several problems including intermittent attacks of gastroenteritis, and having become chairfast she was doubly incontinent and depressed. She was found to have severe onychogryphosis with ulceration, and once this had been dealt with by the chiropodist, she again became fully ambulant, no longer incontinent and able to return home to her husband.

Drug Administration

Drugs are administered at regular intervals throughout the day in accordance with the written instructions of the doctor. Each patient will be following his individual regimen.

Diuretics should always be given early in the day, so that they do not interfere with the patient's rest at night. The nurse should check that the patient has actually swallowed the tablets, as often one finds small bundles hidden in a handkerchief or under the pillows even though the patient was seen to put them in his mouth.

A simple explanation of the action of the tablets often helps, as the patient can see the reason for their administration. One should always, if possible, let the patient take the tablet himself, rather than thrusting it directly into his mouth, which is most unplcasant. Somc tablcts arc largc and difficult to swallow; these can be crushed and mixed with honey. Injections are often unavoidable, and the sites should be rotated so that the patient does not become sore in one spot.

The Patient's Day

As the majority of patients in the unit are up for most of the day, it should be planned for their maximum comfort, so the nurse must ensure they have adequate rest, but also remain fully occupied.

It is general for patients to be up for breakfast. It is not easy for even the most agile person to eat in bed, and impossible for the hemiplegic or otherwise incapacitated patient to do so with ease and comfort. Patients enjoy their meals far more sitting in a chair, and at the same time it eliminates having to feed a number of patients individually.

Everyone should be aided and encouraged to go to the lavatory, and well designed lavatories and sanichairs are an asset. Commodes are often essential for less agile patients, but bedpans rarely need be used.

Dressing should take place in a calm, unhurried atmosphere, as independently as possible, and the staff should be taught to give assistance as and when necessary.

The morning is occupied with visits to the occupational therapy and physiotherapy departments, a bath or shower, a visit from the hairdresser, chiropodist or clergyman.

The nurse should aim at a daily bath for incontinent patients and those with indwelling catheters or a vaginal discharge, and every other day for the rest of the patients. Many have not had a bath for several years, and do not relish the idea when in hospital, but after the first visit are always pleased to go again. The Ambulift has proved invaluable for the nurse and provides a comfortable, safe method of moving the patient in and out of the bath.

The bathroom should be warm and the nurse should take care that the patient does not feel the cold. The water should be kept at 38°C approximately, and plenty of water run in, especially if the Ambulift is used, so that the patient can have a good soak. Towels and clean clothing should all be made available before the bath is begun so that the patient is not kept waiting. Bathing is often a good opportunity for the nurse to have a talk with the patient without interruption.

Showers are also very useful and refreshing for the patient. The elderly patient often seems alarmed at the idea, but having had one once, always seems to enjoy them thoroughly. It is essential that the shower room is very warm, and that the nurse fully understands the thermostat, so that the water is never too hot or too cold.

Lunch served at a communal table can be enjoyed by many, after which some patients like to have an hour's rest on their bed or in a comfortable chair. We have found the Buxton chair ideal for those patients who tend to slide forward out of the ordinary upright varieties; the tipping device prevents slide and enables the patient to have a peaceful rest. An hour in the afternoon may be devoted to some form of group activity, such as bingo, a whist drive, music and movement, painting or the showing of slides. The nursing staff usually take it in turn to organize this and it proves a challenge both for them and for the patients.

Most patients wash their hands and face after tea and are then encouraged to get undressed and retire to bed after supper. By this time they are usually quite tired and ready for a good night's rest, often without the aid of any sedation. Should sedatives be necessary, barbiturates should be avoided, if possible and nitrazepam or chloral hydrate used instead. Barbiturates tend to increase rather than reduce the patient's disorientation and restlessness.

Recording of Nursing Notes

The Kardex system for recording the patient's daily activities and progress is now generally used in most hospitals, and should show at one glance the diagnosis, length of stay, progress and perhaps ultimate goal, i.e. home or residential accommodation. Daily recording is essential, abbreviations should not be used, a full signature should be given and all of the records must be kept for 6–10 years in case reference is required or the hospital should later be sued for negligence regarding some matter.

Care of the Unconscious Patient

During her time in the geriatric unit the nurse will come in contact with the unconscious patient and must be aware of the principles involved in caring for this patient.

The most common cause of unconsciousness in the elderly is following a cerebrovascular accident, due to thrombosis, embolus or haemorrhage. It may occasionally be due to poisoning by gas, drugs or alcohol. Infection may be the cause with resulting septicaemia, encephelitis or meningitis. Other causes include severe myxoedema, diabetes, uraemia, hypothermia, hyperthermia, dehydration and cerebral tumours.

On admission the observations which the doctor will ask the nurse to record will vary according to the cause of unconsciousness. In all cases a record of temperature, pulse, respiration and blood pressure will be required at frequent intervals.

The patient will be nursed on his side, the elderly patient usually being nursed in the lateral position, occasionally in the semi-prone position. He must be well supported so that he cannot roll on to his back causing obstruction of the airway with possible inhalation of secretions. It will be necessary to have near at hand:

Oxygen cylinder and face mask
Suction apparatus
Rubber airway
Mouth gag
Tongue-holding forceps
Tongue depressor

It is most important that the nurse maintains a clear airway at all times by keeping the nostrils clear, removing any false teeth and using the suction apparatus to remove any secretions, sputum or vomit.

The patient should have his position changed 2-hourly, both day and night. As elderly people are particularly prone to pressure sores, it is usually wise to nurse the unconscious patient on a ripple bed from the outset. This, however, does not lessen the need for regular turning by the nurse. Regular turning also helps to lessen the risk of chest complications and enables the nurse or physiotherapist to perform passive movements on all the limbs, thus reducing the risk of contractures. When the patient is at rest, the limbs should be well supported on pillows or foam pads, to prevent areas of skin touching each other.

The nurse will wash the patient regularly, taking special care to dry under the folds of the breasts and in the groins. The mouth will be cleaned regularly and the lips kept moist. The eyes should be bathed routinely with a solution of half-strength normal saline, and kept free from crusts.

As the patient is incontinent, catheterization is usually recommended, unless the patient appears to be regaining consciousness quickly. Regular bowel habit should be encouraged by insertion of glycerine suppositories, or by digital removal of faeces by an experienced nurse. After a few days a regular pattern may evolve without the aid of medication.

Initially the unconscious patient will be given intravenous fluids, the quantity and quality determined by the doctor, depending on the electrolyte balance and the cause of unconsciousness. If there is no rapid improvement in the level of unconsciousness, it is normal to progress to nasogastric feeding, as this provides an easier method for regulating the nutritional intake of the patient. The type of feeds given will be discussed by the doctor, nurse and dietitian, depending on the patient's needs (see Chapter 7).

Nursing the unconscious patient demands skill and patience on the part of the nurse. She must remember that the patient is still an individual even though he may be unable to communicate and the nurse should never discuss his condition or his affairs at the bedside.

4 Common Diseases of Old Age

When caring for patients suffering from the diseases which tend more to occur in old age, the nurse will use basic principles which apply to all patients and which have been discussed in the previous chapter. As in all specialties, a knowledge of all the particular diseases, their causes, symptoms, treatment and any special nursing care must be understood and appreciated by the nurse working in the field of geriatrics.

Arthritis

Rheumatoid Arthritis

Although this is primarily a disease of youth and middle age, it continues throughout life into old age. It can also commence in old age, usually affecting several symmetrical joints, unlike osteoarthrosis which affects 1 or 2 joints and is often asymmetrical.

Cause The cause is unknown. Swelling and joint effusions appear, the joint surfaces become infiltrated, the cartilage breaks up and joint space is lost. Fibrous tissue is laid down around and within the joint. It is a multi-system disease not only causing arthritis but also resulting in systemic signs and symptoms.

Signs and symptoms There is pain, stiffness and swelling of the affected joints and limitation of movement. General malaise, depression, loss of weight, a raised sedimentation rate and tiredness develop. There may be local inflammation with heat and swelling of the joint. In advanced cases a creaking crepitus may be obtained. In severe chronic arthritis the grating sound is caused by the rubbing together of the dried internal surfaces of the joints. There may also be severe wasting of the muscle groups which move the joints.

Treatment This is a disorder of the whole person and therefore a team approach is most important. The aim of treatment is to relieve pain and inflammation and then increase movement so that the patient can lead as active a life as possible without too much discomfort. A balance has to be found between rest and movement. Rest in bed may be necessary at first. The nurse and the physiotherapist must ensure that there is good position of all the joints. Padded splints or light plastic casts may be used. Passive movements may be commenced as soon as possible and eventually the patient will graduate to activities of daily living encouraged by nurse, physiotherapist and occupational therapist. The nurse may find it necessary to encourage an old person to accept a full and varied diet. Many old people living alone tend to make do with bread and butter and cups of tea. The patient may need help with cutting up solid food if the hands are deformed and painful. The doctor will ensure that anaemia and possible vitamin and mineral deficiencies are corrected with the appropriate supplements. Emphasis should be placed upon red meats, milk, eggs and fresh fruit. It is often necessary in hospital to add iron, ascorbic acid, folic acid, multivitamins and calcium to the medication.

Effective analgesia should be given and at regular intervals so that the patient can move without undue discomfort. Paracetamol is preferable to aspirin, which causes gastro-intestinal haemorrhage due to gastric irritation and occasional hypersensitivity.

Steroids may occasionally be used but are not often justifiable for long-term use for the elderly patient. They relieve symptoms only while they are being used and have many side-effects. An intra-articular injection of cortisone to a specific joint, particularly the knee, by the doctor, is usually of great value. There is a dramatic improvement within 36 hours due to the anti-inflammatory effect of the drug, and the improvement may last for several weeks or months. A strict aspetic technique must be used to avoid the introduction of infection. Patients who have severe deformities of the joints after years of suffering from rheumatoid arthritis are often seen in the Geriatric Unit. The patients generally have a low pain threshold. Some help may be given by gentle exercises, possibly preceded by wax baths. Little improvement will be expected in mobility but eventually the patient may be helped by specially designed aids.

Case history Mrs D., aged 78 years, was admitted from home to the Acute Assessment Ward of the Geriatric Unit. She had spent most of her life in Africa, and was a well-known artist, and also had been an adept needlewoman, having been a seamstress by trade. She had developed acute rheumatoid arthritis 6 weeks before admission, affecting mainly her hands, the finger and wrist joints, so that she had poor grip, and she also had muscle tenderness of the left upper arm. She was unable to hold small articles—a needle to sew or a paintbrush for painting. She was a delightful lady, who was very annoyed by her disability and determined to overcome her handicap. She settled well into the ward routine and was most cooperative about her treatment. She started a course of the steroid prednisolone 10 mg per day for a limited period. She had a course of wax baths prior to her physiotherapy which she found most helpful. She also attended the occupational therapy department where she learnt to use her hands again and even managed to start painting. Four weeks later she was discharged from hospital considerably improved, and attended the Day Hospital weekly to ensure that improvement was maintained. After a month she was reviewed by the doctor in the out-patient clinic and her steroid dosage was gradually reduced and was discontinued altogether 4 weeks later.

Osteoarthrosis

This can be described as a degenerative arthritis, to distinguish it from rheumatoid arthritis, since no inflammation occurs; degeneration of the articular cartilage and weight bearing surface of large joints takes place, and may result in shortening of the affected limb. The disease may affect one or several joints, but not, as in rheumatoid arthritis, many joints. The onset is slow; the patient tends to complain of pain some time after onset, and feels tired. The irregular formations of new bone round the joint interferes with movement.

Cause The cause is wear and tear, often aggravated by obesity, but osteoarthrosis can occur following an injury or fracture involving a joint. The common joints affected are the knee, hip and all weight-bearing joints.

Signs and symptoms Pain, stiffness and swelling of the joint occur, and in some cases the joint becomes deformed. The pain is variable, sometimes severe, sometimes minimal. If the hip joint is affected, this is more disabling and continuous pain is usually present radiating to the groin and leg. As the disease progresses there is increasing stiffness and deformity which makes dressing difficult, also rising from a low chair or toilet or getting in or out of the bath. Difficulty may also be experienced when the patient sits up in bed.

Treatment The most important aim is for the patient to lose weight. These people may be more cooperative than usual, as they may realize the necessity for this and benefit from the relief of pain when weight loss is established. Adequate analgesics should be given at regular intervals and regular exercises given by the physiotherapists. For these patients exercises performed where the limbs are swung in rope and sling suspension are of great value. Mobility will be encouraged by the use of sticks, tripod or walking frame.

Surgery has an important part to play in this disease. The common operation is arthrodesis or arthroplasty of the affected joint, arthrodesis being the fixation of a movable joint by surgical operation, arthroplasty involving replacement with a metallic or acrylic prosthesis. Arthrodesis is most commonly performed on the knee and arthroplasty on the hip, although the latter is now being developed for the knee also. The patient who will progress most satisfactorily is the one with severe pain, who is alert and cooperative and has the will and drive to recover, as rehabilitation following surgery is a slow process. At all times the nurses and therapists must strive to prevent the formation of contractures which may prevent the patient achieving maximum mobility.

Case history Mrs L., aged 88 years, was admitted to hospital in early February having taken to her bed after Christmas with influenza. She was a very obese, talkative lady, who lived alone in a converted flat in her nephew's house. As a result of being bedridden and immobile she had become doubly incontinent and had also developed large blisters on both heels. Owing to her obesity and arthritis the home nurse could no longer manage her and the general practitioner asked the geriatrician to call and give his advice. He felt that a period in hospital with active rehabilitation would benefit this lady but was dubious as to whether she would ever return home.

X-ray examination showed her to have severe osteoarthrosis of the right hip and moderate arthritis of the left hip and both knees. She also had painful oedema of both legs due to stasis.

Intensive therapy was begun immediately and although she could not stand initially, it was not long before Mrs L. was dressing herself and taking a few steps with a walking frame. The blisters on her heels were quickly reduced, and the oedema slowly improved with exercise and a mild diuretic. This is an agent, usually a drug, which increases the excretion of urine. Despite the diuretic her incontinence was soon eliminated as she was offered and helped to the commode or lavatory regularly and frequently initially. Soon she came under the additional care of the occupational therapist, who found her unable to cope with pants, stockings and shoes when dressing. Again all these problems were overcome; she was given a stocking garter and shoes with elastic laces. Mrs L. gradually lost weight on her reducing diet, despite a few lapses which were always detectable by the wicked twinkle in her eye!

Three months after admission, it was decided that Mrs L. was fit and able to return home to live alone again, much to her delight. The therapists checked her bed and chair heights at home and saw that there were no difficult stairs to negotiate. She attended the Day Hospital twice weekly, so that her weight could be checked and her mobility maintained.

Non-articular Rheumatism

Many elderly patients complain of pain for which there is no obvious cause. Muscles, ligaments and tendons appear to be involved. The pain is often severe and as a result the affected area tends to become immobile. The areas most commonly affected are the neck, resulting in torticollis (stiff neck), and the shoulder, causing 'frozen shoulder'. Once it has been demonstrated that joint and bone diseases are not the cause of the pain, usually by X-ray, the pain and immobility may respond to gentle exercise and heat.

Osteoporosis

This is a common disease of the elderly, especially women.

Cause It is the result of a reduction in the amount of bone mass without any change in its constitution. The bone becomes more brittle and is liable to bend or fracture. It may be due to a low calcium intake or a failure to absorb calcium. It can result from prolonged inactivity or long-term use of steroids as in rheumatoid arthritis.

Signs and symptoms The main symptom is pain. The disease generally occurs in the spine which becomes bent—kyphosis—and results in loss of height. There may be compression fractures of vertebral bodies.

Treatment Treatment is slow and often unsatisfactory. The calcium intake may be increased in the form of extra milk plus calcium gluconate or calcium lactate daily. Anabolic hormones may help. Intramuscular Durabolin may be given weekly or Deca-durabolin once every 3 weeks. Vitamin D may be supplemented if there is a possibility of vitamin deficiency.

A firm surgical support may be supplied to relieve backache, but unfortunately this may be seldom worn once the patient leaves hospital. Patients require considerable encouragement and explanation to become accustomed to the support and obtain benefit from wearing it.

Case history Miss X., aged 86 years, was admitted from home, no longer able to cope with life, having recently developed severe pain in the dorsal spine. Thus she was unable to move without pain, her arms being especially affected. She could not brush her hair or dress herself and had difficulty feeding and getting out of a chair. An X-ray of the spine revealed extensive osteoporosis with a compression fracture of the fifth and sixth dorsal vertebrae. After consultation with the orthopaedic surgeon a high corset was ordered which did give some support. Adequate analgesia in the form of Distalgesic and ibuprofen was given and her calcium intake was supplemented daily with Calciferol and Calcium-Sandoz, and weekly with injections of Durabolin.

Improvement was slow but steady and after several weeks the pain was considerably reduced, and the patient fairly mobile and quite independent. However, she decided that she would no longer be able to manage entirely alone and would live in residential accommodation organized by the local authority.

Cervical Spondylosis

Cervical spondylosis is a disease of middle or old age and results from degeneration or protrusion of the intervertebral discs.

Signs and symptoms These include tingling of the arms and hands, occurring especially at night. This is caused by disturbance to the nerve roots either by disease or fibrosis. There may also be some weakness and wasting of the arms and radiation of pain to the chest wall, neck or back. In addition the patient may have difficulty in walking and some loss of balance.

Vertebrobasilar insufficiency may also result from cervical

spondylosis where the degenerative changes in the discs of the neck cause shortening and the vertebral arteries become kinked. The patient may suffer from confusion at times, vertigo and transient episodes of loss of consciousness.

Treatment Neck traction is not often tolerated by the elderly and the most pleasant form of treatment is immobilization by means of a light plastic or Plastazoate collar supporting the chin and neck.

Hypertension

Blood pressure is the pressure of the blood within the arteries of the body. With the contraction of the left ventricle, blood is forced into the aorta and then into the large arteries, the small arteries and arterioles. The systolic pressure is the arterial pressure at the height of the pulsation, and the diastolic pressure is the arterial pressure at the lowest level of pulsation. The blood pressure is affected by a decrease in the size of the lumen of the vessel, the constriction of the vessel and deposits within that vessel. It is also dependent on the force of the ventricular contractions.

Blood pressure is usually measured by the auscultatory method. The stethoscope is placed over the brachial pulse, the cuff is pumped until no sound is heard, the artery is collapsed by pressure of the cuff and no blood is flowing through. The cuff is then released and as the blood passes through sounds are heard as the artery collapses and fills. Eventually sounds diminish in intensity as the artery no longer collapses. The diastolic pressure is taken at the point when the sound starts to diminish. In order to obtain an accurate reading, the nurse must remember to have the sphygmomanometer on a level with the patient's arm.

Quite a large proportion of the elderly, particularly women, suffer from hypertension, most commonly essential hypertension of the benign type, which is often associated with obesity. This may progress on to left ventricular hypertrophy and eventually left ventricular failure which is discussed later in this chapter. Hypertensive elderly women, however, tend to adjust without effects other than occasional giddiness and falls. Hypertension may also result in cerebrovascular disease and cerebro-arteriosclerosis which are discussed in Chapter 8.

In cases of obesity, treatment by diet alone may be sufficient if the patient is cooperative. The only hypotensive drugs commonly used in the elderly are methyldopa and thiazide diuretics in small doses, with a strict watch being kept on the patient's blood pressure. Any dizziness or falls should be reported by the nurse to the doctor. If there are no specific symptoms or signs, the doctor may decide that no treatment is necessary.

Cerebrovascular Disease

There are reported to be 100 000–120 000 new cases of cerebrovascular accident every year, and 75% of these occur in the over-65 age group. There is thought to be a 50% survival rate after the first 'stroke'.

Cause There are 3 main causes of cerebrovascular disease.

Cerebral thrombosis This may be due to shock, infection, a sudden fall in blood pressure, leukaemia, polycythaemia or hypoglycaemia. The thrombosis may take place at rest or when sleeping, often extending over hours or days. The onset is gradual with drowsiness, followed by loss of consciousness or a fit. There may be a weakness of one side of the body which if mild is known as hemiparesis, and if severe with paralysis as hemiplegia. Difficulties in speech may occur and, if the brain stem is affected, difficulties in swallowing. The initial damage and signs may improve after a few days when the collateral circulation takes over but residual damage remains.

Cerebral haemorrhage This may be caused by uncontrolled, possibly unsuspected, hypertension. A diastolic pressure of over 110 mmHg in the elderly should be regarded with suspicion. The cerebral haemorrhage may also be caused by a bleeding disorder. The patient is often in a coma on arrival at hospital, and the outcome is frequently fatal. The onset is very sudden, frequently with loss of consciousness, and death may follow rapidly.

Cerebral embolism This most commonly occurs in the patient with atrial fibrillation or bacterial endocarditis. As in cerebral haemorrhage the onset is sudden and the degree of disability is obvious immediately.

Treatment In all cases of cerebrovascular accident, the doctor will assess the patient's ability to breathe, swallow and cough and whether the muscle tone is flaccid or spastic. He will also test his reaction to pain, temperature and touch. He will also look for visual defects such as hemianopia which occurs when there is loss of part of the visual field. The doctor will also note any difficulties with speech. Those which may occur are: aphasia, when there is total absence of speech; dysarthria, when there is a mechanical fault present; and apraxia, when there is a failure to recognize common articles. There will also be assessment of the intellectual and emotional disturbances of the patient. Sometimes there are signs of aggression or depression, difficulty in communication and also lack of motivation. The team of doctors, nurses and therapists will want to know what the patient was like before the stroke occurred, so that they can set themselves a goal, and also a time limit before reassessment is made.

Complications Oedema of the affected limb may develop as the result of stasis. This may affect the hand, foot and ankle, and may be improved by elevation and support. Pressure sores may occur, so frequent change of position and careful protection of vulnerable areas will be necessary. Incontinence may follow a cerebrovascular accident. Contractures may occur if the affected limb is not well supported at all times and both passive and active exercises are given. Emotional lability frequently occurs, causing the patient to be very cheerful at one time and very depressed a few minutes later. Rejection of the affected side may occur when the patient is unable to acknowledge that his limbs are disabled, thus making work very difficult for the physiotherapist. Chest infection is often a common complication following a cerebrovascular accident and is a common cause of death, especially for those patients in coma. Thus wherever possible it is necessary for the patient to be up and as mobile as possible.

General nursing care On admission to the ward, the patient may be nursed in bed for a few days if acutely ill. The nurse will be required to give 2-hourly care of pressure areas, with frequent changing of position, regular mouth care and frequent fluids.

If necessary a board and pillow may be placed at the foot of the bed to give support and prevent footdrop occurring. A bed cradle must always be placed in the bed to prevent pressure from the bedclothes causing sores of the heels and to enable the patient to move his legs freely. If the patient has difficulty in supporting himself in bed, one cot side may be used on the affected side to prevent the patient slipping out of bed (see Fig. 9, p. 48).

Two-hourly toilet training is often necessary if the patient has difficulty passing urine or regaining control. The patient may be sat out on the commode at the same time as the nurse is attending to his pressure areas. Only in very severe cases should a permanent indwelling catheter be necessary.

Physiotherapy will begin almost immediately, and the nurse must work closely with the physiotherapist, so that she can continue with both the active and passive movements. At a later stage, the occupational therapist will also be called in to treat the patient, to help him with the activities of daily living, and to assess whether he will be able to manage at home or may need to go somewhere where more help is available.

If the patient is right-handed and has a right hemiplegia with resulting speech difficulties, the nurse must take particular time and trouble to anticipate his needs and prevent him becoming too frustrated by his problems. The nurse must ensure that the patient's locker is on the correct side of the bed so he can easily reach his possessions. Once the patient starts getting up, he should wear strong shoes and, as soon as he is able, his own clothes, as this has a very good effect on morale. Some of the clothes may need modifying with the help of the occupational therapist. Eventually the patient may need a caliper or some form of support for the leg, but this will only be decided after a reasonable period of intensive treatment, as they are expensive and have to be made individually. The nurse must remember that the patient will still need frequent movement even when sitting in a chair.

The process is slow and improvement is gradual and in these cases the patients will need much encouragement, as they will frequently become despondent and there is a tendency towards dependence on the nursing and other staff. Relatives, too, will need much support from the nursing staff, especially when communication is difficult. It must be explained that progress will be slow and improvement can continue for up to two years.

The prognosis will depend on the length of the period during which the patient is unconscious and the extent of the stroke with its associated defects. It will depend, too, on whether it is the first or subsequent stroke, and the speed with which the patient is admitted to hospital. Finally, the patient's emotional and physical state, and the relatives' attitude and cooperation will have an effect upon the extent of improvement.

Case history Mrs D., aged 68 years, was admitted to hospital from home having had a cerebrovascular accident 3 weeks previously, leaving her with a left hemiplegia. She was a widow and lived alone, but her daughter and young family lived near by. She had made limited progress at home, but the general practitioner and home nurse felt that she would benefit from a period of active rehabilitation in hospital. On admission she was found to have weakness of the left side of her face, leg and arm. She was dysarthric, this being partly due to loose dentures, which were adjusted during her stay in hospital. Dysarthria is difficulty in articulating words as a result of disease of the central nervous system. She was also found not to have had her bowels open for 2 weeks, and this caused considerable discomfort. However, this was quickly remedied with a series of 6 enemas which after careful explanation quite put the patient's mind at rest. Mrs D. was of slight build and great determination. She greatly benefited from help from the physiotherapist, occupational therapist and nurse, progressing from walking with a tripod to a stick before being discharged. Her balance was good on the whole, and this was helped as she was a retired teacher of ballet dancing. She learned to dress herself independently and, before being discharged home after 8 weeks, had practised washing, ironing, washing up, laying the table, cooking and walking outside. She had also bathed herself using a seat bench. All went well after discharge and she continued to visit the Day Hospital twice weekly for 12 weeks, so that she could continue her physiotherapy and occupational therapy. She also attended the old people's club locally of which she was the Queen that year. Eventually Mrs D. was discharged from the Day Hospital 6 months after her original stroke, able to manage entirely alone.

Incipient Congestive Heart Failure

This is a common disability of old age for which there are many causes, the most common being ischaemic heart disease, but including anaemia and occasionally thyrotoxicosis or myxoedema. It may also be precipitated by disease of the lungs such as chronic bronchitis.

Signs and symptoms The most common symptoms are dyspnoea and orthopnoea. A cough is nearly always present. The patient also complains of weakness and lassitude. Many patients become confused and agitated, and suffer from insomnia and nocturnal restlessness due to an inadequate supply of oxygen to the brain. Oedema of the feet and ankles also occurs but this is frequently present in elderly people who do not have heart failure.

Treatment The basic treatment is rest, but this must be assessed with care. The elderly patient is often more comfortable sitting in a chair and the exercise of getting out of bed into the chair helps to preserve mobility. Walking a few steps to the lavatory may also be beneficial. Digitalis is nearly always given in these cases as it slows and strengthens the heart beat, and controls atrial fibrillation which may be present. Old people are often very sensitive to this drug, and the nurse should record the pulse before giving the dosage.

The doctor must be informed if it is abnormally slow or irregular. The normal dose of digoxin is 0·25 mg once or twice daily, but occasionally digoxin P.G. (paediatric/geriatric) may be given 0·0625 mg twice daily, as old people tend to be so sensitive. Digoxin may also cause nausea and vomiting, and if this is so lanatoside (Cedilanid) may be given as an alternative. Sensitivity to digoxin is frequently aggravated by hypokalaemia—low potassium due to diuretics. Diuretics may be needed and the type used may depend upon the patient's ability to control the act of micturition. Frusemide 40–80 mg orally or 40 mg by intramuscular injection gives a rapid result, its action only lasting four hours. Hydrochlorothiazide 25–100 mg has a slower action, and may be more beneficial to those with a tendency to incontinence. It may be necessary to change the diuretic from time to time, as it may cease to be effective. A potassium supplement will be given, as potassium is lost in the urine. Salt restriction is necessary for all patients with heart failure, and in severe cases salt should not be added to the cooking. Unfortunately, most patients with congestive heart failure lack an appetite and this restriction of salt does not help the palatability of food. This type of patient often tends to be dissatisfied and disgruntled and needs much patience and care from the nursing staff.

Myocardial Infarction

This is a common complaint in the elderly person but often presents without any signs or symptoms. Unlike middle-aged patients, who present with pain and shock, the elderly patient may only complain of dizziness, breathlessness and some confusion. Diagnosis may only be confirmed when an electrocardiograph has been performed, and this should be carried out routinely in all elderly patients. The patient is nursed in bed only for the first few days and then is encouraged to be up and using the lavatory, to prevent the formation of deep vein thrombosis and pulmonary embolism. Oxygen may be given initially to relieve dyspnoea. The most comfortable method of administration is by Ventimask allowing the patient to inhale air and oxygen, or via nasal spectacles which fit comfortably into the nostrils. Hypotension is usually present initially and if this is severe the doctor may prescribe intramuscular hydrocortisone or Aramine to raise the blood pressure. Cardiac pain may be relieved by glyceryl trinitrate tablets 0·5–1·0 mg sucked sublingually, i.e. beneath the tongue. Mycardol has a similar effect but is longer acting and is used to prevent pain occurring. The use of anticoagulants, due to difficulty in stabilization, is not generally advocated for the elderly unless there are repeated episodes of infarction or embolism. Drugs known as beta-blockers, such as propanolol or oxypranolol, may also be used in the treatment of cardiac pain and arrhythmias which often cause considerable discomfort to elderly patients.

Anoxic Chest Disease

Acute Bronchitis

This may occur suddenly and unexpectedly in the elderly and often without pyrexia, i.e. a raised temperature. It is a common cause of death especially when associated with severe bronchospasm. The patient presents with a dry cough, wheezing respirations and breathlessness. It occurs mainly in those patients who have a history of chronic bronchitis. The patient should be kept warm, but should be encouraged to get up in a chair quite soon and also to move around. Fluids should be encouraged and these should contain as much nourishment as possible as the patient frequently lacks an appetite. These may include fresh fruit juice, Complan and Carnation breakfast foods.

Chronic Bronchitis

The incidence of this disease is high in the United Kingdom, particularly in the northern industrial areas where the climate is cold and damp. It is also more commonly seen in the obese patient, and those who suffer sudden change in the temperature of their environment from hot to cold. It is aggravated by smoking. In early stages an attack usually follows a cold which develops into bronchitis. Eventually there may be a persistent cough in the winter. Patients are not usually admitted to hospital specifically with chronic bronchitis, and manage to cope at home. They may be given a cough mixture, and bronchial dilators such as salbutamol or Choledyl are used.

Pneumonia

Bronchopneumonia is fairly common in the elderly, especially following bronchitis, cerebrovascular accident, congestive heart failure and fractured femur. It is another very common cause of death. There is often no pyrexia but a tachycardia (abnormally rapid action of the heart) and rise in the respiratory rate. The patient lacks an appetite (anorexia) and may also have a sudden mental disturbance. The patient is usually nursed in bed in the upright position or in a comfortable chair. Regular care of pressure areas must be taken and hygiene maintained. Nourishing fluids are given in the form of fresh fruit juice, Complan and Carnation breakfast foods. An appropriate antibiotic will be prescribed by the doctor, ampicillin being the most common drug of choice, either orally or by intramuscular injection. Care should be taken when giving sedatives, and barbiturates should be avoided. Oxygen should be available if necessary.

Anaemia

This occurs with great frequency among the elderly population for various reasons. The patient presents with pallor, especially of the mucous membranes, breathlessness, palpitations, tiredness, swollen ankles and often confusion. There are three main types, but they may occur in combination.

Iron Deficiency Anaemia

Iron deficiency is the most common cause of anaemia in the elderly, and is due to chronic blood loss from hiatus hernia, carcinoma of the stomach or colon, diverticuli, haemorrhoids, or from taking drugs, e.g. aspirin, which may cause bleeding. Malnutrition and poor absorption of iron can also be a cause.

Symptoms These may be difficult to define if anaemia is of slow onset. Where the haemoglobin falls below 10g/100 ml patients may complain of tiredness, breathlessness on exertion, headaches and lack of concentration. Clinically they may have spoon-shaped or brittle nails, a smooth tongue and cracking at the corners of the mouth, when the haemoglobin has been very low for a considerable time.

Treatment The cause must first be established and the nurse may well be asked to observe the colour of the stools and collect specimens for testing for occult blood. Oral iron is given by choice in the form of ferrous sulphate, ferrous gluconate or slow-release iron. Ascorbic acid is generally given also to elderly people to aid absorption. It is often necessary to give iron intramuscularly. There are two common preparations, Jectofer which is more quickly absorbed, or Imferon of which less is excreted in the urine. The injection is given deep into the muscle of the upper outer quadrant of the buttock to avoid staining the skin. In hospital a total dose infusion of Imferon may be given intravenously over a period of 8 hours. The nurse should observe the patient for a reaction which may occur within a few minutes of the infusion, commencing with pyrexia, headache, dizziness, sweating and loin pain. The doctor should be informed and the infusion discontinued immediately. It may be necessary to give 0·5 ml of intramuscular adrenaline 1:1000.

Vitamin B12 Deficiency

Addisonian or pernicious anaemia is seen most commonly in persons of white races over 60 and in about two-thirds of those affected there is a familial history. It is caused by achlorhydria in the stomach preventing the absorption of vitamin B12.

Symptoms The patient may not be seen in hospital until the symptoms are severe, as the anaemia develops slowly and the patient adapts to this. There may be soreness of the tongue, a lemon or yellow tinge to the skin and the patient may complain of tingling and numbness of the hands and feet. Heart failure may also develop due to anoxia of the heart muscle. The nurse may be asked to help with the diagnosis by performing a histamine test meal or Diagnex Blue test which measures the amount of acid in the stomach.

Treatment Replacement therapy is necessary by giving the patient intramuscular 1000 μg cyanocobalamin initially daily or weekly depending upon the severity of the anaemia and eventually monthly for the rest of the patient's life.

Case history Mrs Y., aged 84 years, was admitted to hospital from home. She had recently flown over from South

Africa to spend a holiday with her daughter. She had tended to become rather tired for some time and shortly after her arrival in England she noticed her ankles were swelling, and she became breathless, especially after climbing stairs. These are classical signs of heart failure. She also had lost some weight and suffered from loss of appetite. She visited the general practitioner who took a haemoglobin estimation and found it to be 4·29 g/100 ml. Consequently he recommended her to spend a short period in hospital for full investigation. Her blood results showed iron deficiency and B12 deficiency, her serum B12 being undetectable whereas the normal level is 140–500 μg/100 ml of blood. She was given a course of daily Jectofer injections for two weeks, and cyanocobalamin 1000 μg on alternate days for one week and then weekly. After one month her haemoglobin had risen to 8·9 mg/100 ml and Mrs Y. had lost much of her lassitude and pallor, and her appetite had improved. Her heart failure was no longer evident, her swollen ankles and breathlessness having disappeared. Mrs Y. was discharged back to continue her visit to her daughter and the home nurse was asked to call monthly now to give her her cyanocobalamin injection. She was seen in the out-patient department two weeks later, her haemoglobin having risen to 11·49 mg/100 ml and she was feeling very fit indeed. Six weeks later she flew home to South Africa, feeling she had really benefited from her visit to England although it had not been quite as she had expected!

Folic Acid Deficiency

Folic acid is also necessary for the development of the red blood corpuscles. It is found in liver and green vegetables. Anaemia due to folic acid deficiency is often accompanied by vitamin B12 deficiency in elderly people. The signs and symptoms are similar and treatment is by replacement therapy. The normal dose of folic acid is 5 mg 3 times daily, as tablets. Before treatment is commenced the serum folate level should be estimated by the biochemical laboratory, and this should be repeated after the course of treatment.

Mature Onset Diabetes

This is common in a mild form in many elderly people usually commencing in the sixth decade.

Signs and symptoms These are less obvious than in younger patients who develop diabetes mellitus, as the onset is slow. Some cases are only suspected after a routine ward urine test and diagnosed by taking a blood sugar or when a glucose tolerance test is performed showing a diabetic curve. The patient may complain of polyuria (frequency of passing urine even during the night) and polydypsia (thirst). He may have a change of bowel habit and loss of weight. If he sustains an injury, he finds it takes some time to heal. Although the onset of diabetes is more gradual in the elderly, as the disease may have been present for some years undetected, complications are more frequently seen; peripheral vascular disease may occur with resulting gangrene and there may be diabetic neuropathy and ocular disorders which include disorders of the retina and the formation of cataracts.

Treatment Many patients may be treated by the control of diet alone. The nurse should explain the importance of the diet to the patient and make sure that the patient understands which foods are allowed and which must only be taken in limited quantities. The dietician should also visit the patient before he is discharged from hospital, to make sure that all is understood, and if necessary should also see the relatives.

Patients who are obese because their carbohydrate intake is too high will need a great deal of encouragement to persuade them to give up the foods they enjoy. If they are pensioners there may be financial difficulties in addition, since many protein foods are expensive—meat, for example.

When the patient is admitted with a very high blood sugar and with ketones present in the urine due to excess fat being burned to produce energy, control must commence with insulin, given by injection. Although soluble insulin several times daily may be required initially, eventually it may only be necessary to give a slow-acting insulin daily. Drugs given orally may be sufficient to control the disease, these include tolbutamide, chlorpropramide and phenformin. During this time it is necessary for the nurse to test the patient's urine 4-hourly and record the results, so that the doctor can adjust the treatment accordingly. The patient, or a relative, must be taught how to test urine, and also give insulin if necessary.

Hypoglycaemia may occur and both patient and nurse should be aware of the signs and treatment. It is most likely to be avoided when the patient is well controlled, it is always better to have a little glycosuria than to risk hypoglycaemia. If hypoglycaemia does occur, the patient becomes very confused, starts to sweat and complains of feeling faint and dizzy. If treated promptly, it is only necessary to give a drink containing 20 g of glucose or to give 2 or 3 lumps of sugar if the patient is at home. If it is too late for this treatment and the patient is momentarily unconscious, 20–30 ml of intravenous dextrose 50% may be given by the doctor. Mild hypoglycaemic attacks should always be reported to the doctor and noted on the diabetic chart, as a change in treatment is probably indicated. Since the complication of peripheral vascular disease is fairly common in the elderly, sometimes with resulting gangrene, the nurse must pay particular attention to washing and drying the patient's feet. Care should be taken when cutting the toenails, and the patient should be referred to the chiropodist if necessary. The patient should be told the importance of this care, so that it will be continued at home. Domiciliary chiropody, when it is necessary, is arranged through the Area Health Authority.

Case history Miss M., aged 76 years, was admitted from home with a history of loss of weight, loose stools, frequency of urine and thirst for 2–3 months. Several weeks before she had also damaged her foot when she tripped over a stone in the garden, and this small lesion had failed to heal. She was sent in to hospital by her general practitioner who thought that she had a possible malignant growth of the colon on account of the recent bouts of diarrhoea and loss of weight. Routine ward urinalysis on admission showed a 2% glycosuria and this gave an immediate clue to her true diagnosis. The blood sugar proved to be 408 mg/100 ml. She was given 120 g carbohydrate diet, as Miss M. had a good appetite and was certainly not overweight. She was stabilized on a sliding scale of soluble insulin, and then controlled by a dose of chlorpropramide aided by phenformin. Throughout this time routine 4-hourly urinalysis was recorded and after stabilization she only occasionally had mild glycosuria, and the sore on her foot began to heal. Within 8 weeks she was discharged home to live alone. She fully understood her diet and had written to the British Diabetic Association to obtain some special diabetic recipes. After 2 or 3 uneventful months Miss M. became generally unwell with a urinary tract infection, and took to her bed. As there was no one to look after her at home she was readmitted to hospital. When she arrived she was found to have a gangrenous area on the left heel. Following an appropriate antibiotic the urinary tract infection cleared, but the heel failed to respond to treatment and her glycosuria became erratic and difficult to control because of the presence of infection, thus requiring her once again to be controlled by a sliding scale of insulin. The condition of her heel rapidly deteriorated and eventually a below-knee amputation was performed by the surgeons.

Miss M. recovered well and within 6 weeks a prosthesis had been fitted, and she was walking well. Eight weeks later she was discharged to a convalescent home, eventually to enter residential accommodation, as she herself felt unable to cope alone again at home.

Hyperthyroidism

This is not an uncommon disease of the elderly although the patient does not usually present with all the signs and symptoms that would be found in a young person suffering from thyrotoxicosis.

Signs and symptoms Not all patients have an obvious goitre or exophthalmos, which is abnormal protrusion of the eyeballs, nor indeed an increased appetite. However, many do have tachycardia with atrial fibrillation, loss of weight and a tremor. This is not a positive sign, as many elderly people do have a tremor unrelated to thyrotoxicosis. When investigating the patient with thyrotoxicosis the nurse will be asked to keep an accurate record of the patient's weight and to record a sleeping pulse rate. A rate of over 80 beats per minute may be diagnostic. The doctor will take blood for estimation of the serum protein bound iodine, the normal being in the range of 5·7 mg/100 ml of blood. An iodine-uptake test with measurement of the radioactive iodine excretion in the urine may also be carried out. Treatment may be by methyl or propyl thiouracil or carbimazole, but the nurse must be aware of the side-effects of the latter, which include fever, skin rashes and leucopenia. Surgery is not usually advocated for the elderly. If there is a failure to respond to drugs or side-effects are apparent, or if heart disease is present, the drug of choice is radioactive iodine, because malignant changes which may take place in the gland much later need not be considered.

Case history Miss X., aged 76 years, was seen in the out-patient clinic complaining of loss of weight and diarrhoea. She had gone to see her general practitioner and on examination was also discovered to have swollen ankles, a tachycardia of 120 beats per minute with atrial fibrillation and mild heart failure. She was very agitated, had a tremor of the tongue and hands and an enlarged thyroid was palpable. The doctor found her protein bound iodine to be 16·6 μg, and referred her to the geriatric unit for treatment. She was admitted to hospital for 3 weeks for stabilization and final investigation. Her sleeping pulse was 96–100 beats per minute every night; during the day she was overactive, agitated and had episodes of feeling very flushed and sweating excessively. After all investigations had been completed, she commenced a course of carbimazole. She gradually calmed down, the pulse rate settled and her weight steadied. After 3 weeks she was discharged home, where she lived with her sister, and was subsequently seen regularly in the out-patient department. She continued to improve and gain weight.

Hypothyroidism

This is frequently seen in the elderly although true myxoedema rarely occurs. Occasionally this condition is seen following overactive treatment of hyperthyroidism. It is far more common in women than men.

Signs and symptoms These are often missed and may be attributed merely to old age. They may take several years to develop and the patient and close relatives may not notice them. The patient may become forgetful and hypothermic, when the body temperature becomes considerably lowered, and eventually may go into myxoedemic coma. He may become confused and even psychotic in behaviour, this being known as myxoedema madness. The patient may also complain of tiredness, intolerance of the cold, a dry skin and gain in weight. He may also suffer from constipation. Further signs and symptoms are cramp at night and unsteadiness when walking, deep or hoarse voice and slow speech. The nurse will again be required to make regular recordings of the weight and temperature to ensure that no hypothermia is present. The pulse may be slow. A protein bound iodine estimation will be necessary and serum cholesterol level will be raised.

Treatment This is in the form of replacement therapy by giving thyroid extract or L-thyroxine sodium orally, in small doses initially and gradually increasing the dose. Response takes about 10 days. The sudden stimulation of the body processes may throw an extra strain on the heart, and care must be taken to avoid this. Those patients who lapse into coma are fortunately very rare and very few recover. The coma usually occurs during the winter and the patient may have an added infection. Occasionally he recovers from the coma and dies shortly afterwards in heart failure.

Case history Mrs D., aged 86 years, was admitted from home where she lived with her daughter. She had gradually become more confused and had begun to fall about, making her unsafe to leave alone. As both her son-in-law and daughter were out all day, it was decided to seek a hospital bed. On admission to hospital Mrs D. had dry, coarse skin and hair, she was disorientated and inclined to wander and on one or two occasions when she managed to go about unsupervised she did in fact fall. She admitted to gaining weight and had a rather hoarse voice and slow speech. A protein bound iodine estimation was sent to the laboratory and was found to be only 3·2 μg. Treatment was begun with 0·05 mg tablets of L-thyroxine twice daily. After 10 days improvement was noted, and this continued gradually and steadily. After 3 weeks the confusion had cleared, and the patient became an active, mobile member of the ward showing every consideration to other patients. A week later she was discharged home to live with her family and was followed up as an out-patient.

Hypothermia

This occurs if the body temperature falls below 35°C (95°F). The incidence of hypothermia may vary according to the catchment area of the geriatric unit. Factors influencing the incidence include: (*a*) exposure to cold: prolonged exposure of an inadequately clad and immobile body to a low temperature, e.g. a fall on a cold night on the way to the lavatory;

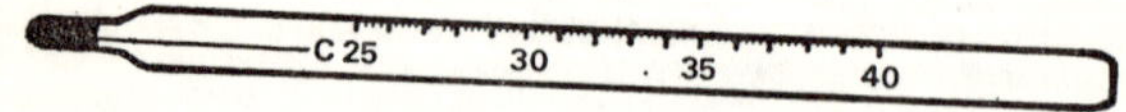

FIG. 11. A low-reading thermometer.

(*b*) defective insulation; (*c*) defective metabolism, hypothyroidism; (*d*) impaired thermoregulatory reflexes, may occur lying in bed if the heat regulating mechanism, centred in the lower part of the brain, is damaged by a cerebrovascular disease; (*e*) drugs and poisons, e.g. chlorpromazine, barbiturates, imipramine or alcohol.

Associated diseases include cerebrovascular disease, hypothyroidism, renal disease and fractures.

Signs and symptoms The patient feels cold, especially over the abdomen. The hands and face are puffy, resembling myxoedema in appearance; there may be ataxia, slurred husky speech, muscular tremor and rigidity. There may be a slow pulse with hypotension and a slow circulation. Respirations are slow and shallow, and pneumonia, although often not evident at first, may quickly develop.

Treatment If the body temperature is above 32°C (90°F) there is no specific treatment. If it is below 31°C (89°F) the patient should be warmed very slowly and not directly, usually by a warm air heater. The majority of patients reach normal temperature in 12 hours, but often rapidly develop pneumonia. The patient will be given antibiotics to cover this eventuality. Corticosteroids may also be given to maintain the circulation. Some fluids may be given by the intravenous route initially, and as soon as the patient is able, nourishing fluids such as fruit juices, meat extracts, Complan and Carnation breakfast foods will be given orally.

Case history Miss M., aged 86 years, was seen at home in November by the geriatrician after an urgent request from the general practitioner. She had developed slurred speech a week previously but had continued to be independent. Her sister had bidden her 'goodnight' the previous evening and all had seemed well. That morning she had gone into the bedroom to find Miss M. in a stuporose condition and unable to speak. When the doctor examined her he found her cyanosed and the abdomen very cold. Her temperature recorded on a low reading thermometer was 31°C (89°F). Her pulse was 60 per minute, the arms and legs were spastic and there was gross oedema up to the thighs. The face was puffy and oedematous also. There were crepitations in the bases of both lungs and mild bronchospasm. The patient was admitted that day to hospital, where she was slowly warmed but unfortunately died two days later from broncho-pneumonia.

Parkinsonism

The types of parkinsonism seen in the geriatric unit affecting the basal ganglia of the brain are arteriosclerotic parkinsonism and 'paralysis agitans' or Parkinson's disease, which usually develops in middle life and progresses on to old age. It is occasionally due to the phenothiazine group of drugs.

Signs and symptoms There is akinesia, an abnormal absence or reduction of muscular movement caused by paralysis of the motor nerves resulting in difficulty in initiating voluntary movement. Tremor occurs unpreceded by any other symptom. It affects resting muscles and may initially affect only one upper limb. It is absent during sleep and is greatly exacerbated by anxiety. It may also be halted by voluntary movement of the affected limb. Rigidity often appears in the early stages of the disease in the form of severe cramp, and then develops into a resistance to passive movement either constant 'lead pipe' or intermittent 'cog wheel'. Associated symptoms may include dysphagia, i.e. difficulty in swallowing, and general flexion in posture including neck and shoulders, arms and hands. The patient also tends to have a staring expression of the eyes, emphasized by the reduction in the rate of blinking. There is a characteristic gait caused by a combination of rigidity, akinesia and associated difficulty in balance. The patient moves by short steps, accelerating as if trying to keep up with his centre of gravity, with the arms kept to the sides instead of swinging.

Treatment These patients need much sympathy and understanding. They have many problems which require a great deal of encouragement and ingenuity on the part of the staff. They may remain mentally alert and be well aware of their physical disability. Drugs and physiotherapy are of much importance. The drugs used fall into two groups. Firstly those of the anticholinergic group such as orphenadrine and benzhexol. Side-effects are confusion, forgetfulness, difficulty with concentration, giddiness and loss of balance. Also, blurring of vision, dry mouth, nausea, tachycardia, difficulty with micturition leading to retention particularly in men, and constipation may occur. Amantidine may also be used in conjunction with two other drugs. L-Dopa is now fairly frequently used in carefully selected cases. It is commenced in small doses and gradually increased and the nurse must know and be able to report to the doctor any side-effects which may occur. The main side-effects include gastrointestinal disorders, anorexia, nausea and vomiting which occurs in about 40% of cases. This may be alleviated if the drug is given with food in the middle of the meal. Other side-effects include hypotension, so the nurse must record a daily blood pressure; psychological abnormalities may also occur, e.g. depression, abnormal voluntary movements and paranoia when the patient may become hostile to his environment together with experiencing relevant delusions. It may be necessary for the doctor to adjust the dose if any of these side-effects occur. The introduction of Sinemet (a combination of levodopa and carbidopa) has reduced many of the side-effects.

Physiotherapy and occupational therapy play a very large part in the treatment of these patients. The physiotherapist will give daily exercises to help the problems caused by the rigidity and akinesia. The occupational therapist will assist the patient with the activities of daily living and all the problems that these involve. She will advise him on the most suitable clothes to wear and even adjust some of the patient's own clothes to make them more manageable. She will also assist with any feeding problems which occur.

Surgery by stereotactic procedures may be used, especially when tremor is severe and unilateral and it may also help rigidity. However it is not often adopted in this age group.

Case history Mrs E., aged 84 years, was admitted from residential accommodation where she had been living very happily for some time. On admission to the home she had been quite mobile and independent, but had recently become bedfast with mild periods of confusion. When seen by the geriatrician, she had a Parkinson facies and a positive globellar tap. She had a festinating gait, i.e. an involuntary quickened gait with a tremor of her left arm only and minimal rigidity. The doctor thought it best to admit her to hospital for a period of intensive physiotherapy and occupational therapy and control of drugs. On admission she was very shy, depressed and immobile. She tended to be incontinent as a result of her immobility and dislike of being a nuisance. However, Mrs E. soon settled into the ward and began to feel happier. She had daily physiotherapy and so began walking slowly with her walking frame. She also attended the occupational therapy department and assisted with dressing, washing and also daily living activities such as washing up, cooking and ironing. Meanwhile, the doctor commenced L-dopa therapy, the nurse noting if any signs of hypotension, confusion and nausea occurred, which in fact they did not. The drug was always given in the middle of a meal. Six weeks later Mrs E. was discharged back to the home fully mobile and independent on 2 g L-dopa daily, and orphenadrine 50 mg three times a day. Eighteen months later the patient was still visiting the out-patient department regularly. She was fully mobile and walking independently.

Postural Hypotension

In elderly people, a sudden drop in blood pressure may occur when they make a sudden change of position from sitting or lying to standing, resulting in giddiness, light headedness and even in momentary loss of consciousness. These people generally are prone to hypotension or have a rather labile blood pressure, and the nurse should record the blood pressure with the patient both lying and standing.

Treatment If a patient suffers from this complaint it is necessary for the nurse to explain to him that he must take time in getting out of bed, rising slowly; similarly, when he has been sitting in a chair, he should get out of the chair slowly. It may also be helpful for the patient to apply crêpe bandages or elastic stockings before getting up in the morning.

Neoplastic Disease

Neoplastic disease is relatively common in the elderly, especially carcinoma of the breast, stomach, colon, prostate gland, skin, lungs and bones. Age is not generally a contra-indication to surgery, provided the patient has no other serious disease. The surgeon will operate on the elderly patient in order to relieve distressing symptoms and enable the patient to lead as active a life as possible and not to be a burden on the relatives. Much depends on the patient's physical ability and his outlook and attitude to life, and also that of the relatives. Radiotherapy and chemotherapy may play a part in treatment, although many neoplasms in the elderly are not radiosensitive. Courses of chemotherapeutic treatment are long, often with unpleasant side-effects, and again are not suitable in this age group, except in selected cases.

Multiple Pathology

It is rare for a patient to be admitted to the geriatric unit with only one disease or disorder. Those elderly who live at home have an average of 3 disorders, and those who come into hospital may have 4 or 5 disorders. Each disease is not lethal by itself, but throws a strain on other systems, the accumulative effect causing disability. Acute illness superimposed upon a chronic disability leads to breakdown and crisis. Frequently the patient admitted with severe osteoarthrosis of the hips for a period of rehabilitation, may have anaemia due to poor absorption of iron and vitamin B12 and also osteoporosis of the spine. In addition to this he may have haemorrhoids causing considerable discomfort, poor sight such as presbyopia, i.e. natural changes that take place in the eyes with advancing age affecting the power of accommodation and resulting in poor sight, which can be improved with new glasses, and presbycussis, i.e. excessive wax in the ear resulting in poor hearing. Hence it can be seen that it is necessary for every patient to have a thorough clinical examination on admission including routine blood tests for haemoglobin, white blood count, erythrocyte sedimentation rate, electrolytes, chest X-ray, urine test and culture, weekly weighing and electrocardiogram.

Falls

Falls are common for the elderly and are often a cause of admission to hospital, and delay the patient's progress when in hospital through injury or loss of confidence. Many can be prevented, although falls are to be expected when advocating and encouraging independence. Patients especially prone to falls are taught how to fall, and how to stand up again unaided if necessary. The most common result is fracture of the upper end of the femur. There are three common causes of falls:

1. *Loss of consciousness.* This group includes patients with transient cerebral ischaemic attacks or those who have small infarcts due to cerebral emboli, and also those with a vertigo or syncope which may be due to a tranquillizer or the sudden onset of anaemia, and those with postural hypotension. Into this group also come those patients with epilepsy, which often presents in the hemiplegic patient or patient with multiple 'small strokes'.

2. *Loss of balance.* This affects those patients with parkinsonism, cerebral arteriosclerosis with shuffling gait and ataxia, i.e. failure of muscle coordination which is usually due to diseases of the cerebellum including vertebrobasilar artery insufficiency. Included in this group are those patients suffering from the effect of certain drugs or overdosage of drugs which should be noted by the nurse. Those to be especially observed are certain tranquillizers, hypertensive drugs, L-dopa and many types of night sedation which may cause the patient to become confused and lose balance when rising at night. Also included in this group are those patients who suffer from cough syncope or micturition syncope. This is caused by transitory cerebral anaemia due to the effect of straining and the latter is particularly common in elderly men with enlarged prostate, the syncope generally occurring at night when the patient gets up to commode or lavatory.

3. *Tripping.* This group is the most preventable and the nurse can do much to overcome and eradicate these falls. The fall may be due to poor sight and therefore there should be good illumination with no deep shadows, especially on stairs and steps. Loose door mats and unnecessary rugs should be removed. Footwear should be examined, and the patient

encouraged to wear leather or rope-soled shoes which give good support. Slippers may be abandoned. Night sedation should be reduced, with no barbiturates; chloral or chloral derivatives only given. For every patient optimum fitness and mobility should be achieved so that falls are reduced to a minimum.

Fractured Femur

Patients are frequently seen following treatment of a fractured femur in the orthopaedic ward, when they progress to the geriatric unit for rehabilitation. It must be remembered that the fracture is often the cause and not the result of the fall. A fracture may occur if the patient turns suddenly, for example when his name is called, no matter how carefully, when the bones are osteoporotic. There are two main types of fracture: subcapital, which is unsatisfactory to treat and is followed by a 40% morbidity, and intratrochanteric, which is far more satisfactory to treat with better results being achieved. The problems involved are the effects of the local injury, the general problems of the elderly in hospital and those caused by the patient having to undergo a general anaesthetic followed by a period of immobility. Complications which may arise are pneumonia, pressure sores, urinary tract infection and uraemia, pulmonary embolisms and deep vein thrombosis. The intratrochanteric fracture may be treated with a pin and plate, and the subcapital fracture by removal of the head of the femur and insertion of a prosthesis. This is a larger operation with a high mortality rate. Complications may result in the prosthesis burrowing into the pelvis or becoming dislocated.

Because of the problems of a general anaesthetic in the elderly, some successful experiments have been undertaken by immediate pinning under local anaesthetic, with the patient up and walking straight away, and being discharged from hospital after 48 hours. It must be remembered that a fractured femur is one of the hazards of progress in the care of the elderly, encouraging their mobilization and independence. However, this is far outweighed by the numerous ill effects following prolonged bed rest and over protectiveness. The increasing problem of the fractured femur in the elderly female has prompted the development of combined geriatric/orthopaedic wards.

Polypharmacy

The danger of improper use of drugs by the elderly is far greater at home where there may be no supervision. Although overdoses of drugs may be taken, it is just as likely that medication may be omitted altogether. Night sedation may be a danger as the dose may be repeated if the patient wakes in the night. The old should have simplified drug schedules with clearly labelled containers. Many practise self-medication with favourite remedies often unknown to their medical advisers. The nurse can do much to help the doctor regulate the dosage and note any side-effects such as vomiting, nausea, loss of balance, falls, dizziness, excessive drowsiness and confusion.

5 The Incontinent Patient

Incontinence is the failure to control the evacuation of the bladder and/or bowels. It is generally associated with geriatric patients and the nurse gives it little consideration until she begins to work on geriatric wards where 30% of the patients are found to be incontinent at some time during their stay. 40% are known to be incontinent in the first week after admission to hospital, and in the long-stay wards 50% remain incontinent.

The problem of incontinence provides a tremendous challenge for the nursing staff. The way in which this is tackled and the general attitude towards the problem is all-important in helping to improve the situation. If the nurse is able to provide a calm, relaxed atmosphere, all patients will be greatly relieved and helped. Scolding, expressions of annoyance and comments passed by the staff are pointless and can only have a detrimental effect on the patient.

Rigid bedpan and commode rounds should not be strictly adhered to and the patient should be encouraged to visit the lavatory whenever he feels the necessity. Keeping the patients active and out of bed will help relieve the situation, and the importance of wearing their own clothes including underwear must be stressed here, as this will raise the morale of the ward and lower the incidence of incontinence. However, often a patient's pleasure at wearing his own clothes will be spoilt if he feels that too much extra work is involved, but once this hurdle has been overcome, the results are usually worthwhile. These difficulties may be offset by a suitably sited launderette either in the Unit or Day Hospital.

Incontinence in the home may be the final factor in producing a crisis which forces the relatives to find accommodation for their elderly person elsewhere. The elderly may seek to disguise their inability to control bladder or bowel function and not infrequently may hide their soiled clothing, causing considerable distress to themselves and to the relatives with whom they are living. Ignorance of the help that can be obtained for incontinent patients and their families is still very prevalent among the general public. Laundry services can be made available by many Local Authorities. There are a variety of plastic pants and pads obtainable for those with only occasional incontinence, and there are several types of disposable sheets, some with a 'one-way' covering so that the patient's skin is not in contact with damp material, e.g. the Polyweb sheet. The Easinurse Mattress on a specially adapted bed has its uses for the mentally alert but immobile patient, as it has a hole in the middle for a receiver, and provided the patient is positioned correctly, may stay dry for some time. For the immobile man it is often adequate to leave in position a urinal which may be fitted with a non-spill valve (Plate VI) but for those who are up and ambulant, there are various types of condom available which attached to rubber tubing, drain into a bag attached to the leg. Clothing is important, as previously stressed, and there are various specialities available too—short vests, washable Terylene trousers, trousers with Velcro openings, dresses with a split down the back and an overlapping skirt.

Incontinence must be viewed objectively as a disability which can be investigated, treated and in most cases alleviated in one way or another.

The nurse plays the most important part in the management of incontinence and in order that she can carry out her work effectively, she must understand some of its causes.

Mechanisms of Normal Control and of Incontinence

Normal micturition occurs when nervous impulses from the stretched muscle wall of the bladder travel to the sacral cord, and impulses travel via the parasympathetic nervous system to the bladder causing the muscle to contract and the sphincter to relax. In the healthy person this is also governed by impulses from the brain transmitted via the sympathetic nervous system, so that the bladder is emptied at a convenient time in the right place. The normal healthy person does not consider the many actions involved in the simple act of micturition.

The elderly person may not completely fill or empty the bladder and uninhibited contractions may occur during the filling and emptying. The elderly also tend to suffer from urgency and precipitancy resulting in 'accidents'. A further complication may be found in nocturia when there is sometimes a reversal of the normal habit and more urine is passed at night than during the day. In addition to these problems there is an overall incidence of urinary infection in old age, which is as high as 20% in those coming into hospital.

Urgency, precipitancy and nocturia tend to precipitate incontinence on admission to hospital owing to an accumulation of factors—strange surroundings, reluctance to ask to go to the lavatory, and the distance that has to be travelled to get there, many patients being accustomed to having a commode by their bed or chair at home.

Urinary Incontinence

There are two main types of incontinence—transitory and established.

Transitory Incontinence

Transitory incontinence is a very common reason for admission to hospital, or recurs very soon after admission. It may occur with the onset of an acute illness such as pyrexia of unknown origin, pneumonia, urinary tract infection or a cerebrovascular accident and is usually accompanied by an acute confusional state, which may only last a few days. Transitory incontinence may occur in the patient with a chronic disability who may not be able to reach a lavatory or commode easily and, lacking motivation at home, lapses into incontinence.

Case history One lady aged 83 years, admitted from such a home, suffered from obesity and osteoarthrosis of the knees, making her immobile. She lived alone, except for a dearly loved, but also incontinent, poodle. She lived in a pleasantly appointed house, which had belonged to her mother, who had died 10 years previously, and who had looked after her daughter overindulgently. During the past year the daughter had become neglected and recently incontinent of urine due to lack of mobility and motivation, so much so that when the social worker visited after admission to hospital, even the floor boards were found to be saturated with urine. After a period of active rehabilitation and training in hospital, this lady was discharged to residential accommodation, mobile and fully continent.

Cause Some patients react to change of environment by abnormal behaviour patterns with an episode of incontinence due to the disruption of their independence by illness, drugs or social factors. Removal to hospital, to relatives or into a home, causing anxiety and fear and even resentment, all may result in a short period of incontinence. Patients may develop a rebellious attitude and feel aggressive at having had to lose their independence and make an unwelcome move, and may also feel neglected by their family. Incontinence may also be a move to seek attention or a reaction to loss of identity.

However, provided there is a calm atmosphere within the ward and the nursing staff adopt a firm but understanding attitude, this period may only last a very short time.

The patients are encouraged by wearing their own clothes which improves their morale, ensures that loss of identity does not take place, and increases their general awareness of themselves and their respectability, thereby retaining their individuality and dignity. The nurse at all times should call them by their correct surname and not by some endearing or childish term.

It has been shown in various surveys of elderly people that 20–30% suffer from urinary tract infection and this again may lead to precipitancy and even transient incontinence. The cause may be stagnating urine in the bladder due to prostatic enlargement in the male, cystocele or damage at spinal cord or cerebral level. The infection usually enters via the urethra and may in the elderly female be also due to inexpert wiping after emptying the bowel, or wearing soiled clothing.

The elderly patient, like a child, may have no signs or symptoms, and yet an infection superimposed on multiple pathology, may tip the balance from independence or semi-independence to complete dependence and crisis, with the patient becoming confused, ill and depressed or bedfast. The usual manifestations of infection may be present, such as fever, rigors, sweating, dysuria, frequency and pain over the bladder or kidneys.

Treatment Before treatment starts a mid-stream specimen of urine should be collected so that the infection may be treated by the appropriate antibiotic. This should be a routine procedure for all patients admitted to the ward, as the incidence of urinary tract infection is very high in the elderly. The specimen should be collected in a sterile receiver, the external genitalia having previously been washed and then swabbed with Savlon solution. If the patient is fully co-operative and ambulant, the specimen may be collected in the lavatory; for the less ambulant and less able it is easiest to collect this whilst the patient is sitting on the commode. For those who are severely disabled or confused, catheterization may be necessary, provided it is carried out under aseptic conditions. The specimen should be sent to the laboratory as soon as possible after it has been obtained, if not, stored in a refrigerator. The most common organisms in the infected urinary tract are the bacteria *Escherichia coli*, *Proteus* and *Paracolon*. The *Klebsiella* organism is now more commonly found in the urine of elderly patients.

The nurse must remember that antibiotics may have unpleasant side-effects and these should be observed. Sulphonamides and nitrofurantoin may both cause skin rashes and the latter also causes stomach upsets and, rarely, peripheral neuropathy. All forms of penicillin may cause allergic reactions and, if given orally for long periods, diarrhoea. Usually acute infections can be treated with one week's course of antibiotics, and the urine should be checked a few days after this is completed.

Fluids must be encouraged and an intake of at least 2 litres a day achieved. This may be difficult as elderly women particularly are very loath to drink if incontinence is feared. As a general rule these patients will avoid fluids even if placed within easy reach. One must also remember to consider the general nutrition of the patient and ensure that he has an adequate intake of calories, vitamins and protein particularly.

When the patient has recovered, the nurse must supervise personal hygiene, ensuring that the patient has frequent baths and that the perineum is properly cleansed after defaecation.

Faecal impaction may be a cause of transitory urinary

incontinence and this must not be overlooked. Overloading of the sigmoid colon and rectum in impaction may obstruct the bladder and impair control, perhaps leading to retention with overflow and urinary incontinence. This situation usually improves once the impaction has been treated.

Established Incontinence

Established incontinence is present in patients who are not acutely ill and continues during their rehabilitation. There are several causes.

1. Structural abnormalities of the bladder and its outlet, e.g. enlargement of the prostate gland, prolapse of the uterus and formation of a cystocele, bladder calculus or carcinoma.

2. Abnormalities concerning the nerve supply to the bladder at spinal cord level or below, e.g. cord tumours, multiple sclerosis, tabes dorsalis and subacute combined degeneration of the spinal cord.

3. Defects in the brain such as those that occur following strokes, cerebral tumours and cerebral arteriosclerosis. Disease of the nerve supply results in three types of neurogenic bladder. (*a*) Increased bladder tone or spastic type of bladder causing urgency and decrease in volume leading to frequency. This situation arises when cortical control is interrupted by organic brain disease. (*b*) Decrease in bladder tone or atony when the sensory nerve supply is damaged. Motor stimulation does not occur resulting in a large residual urine with overflow incontinence. (*c*) Disease or injury of the spinal cord will result in a lower centre for control. The small hypertonic bladder will act independently and frequently resulting in the automatic bladder.

The hyperexcitable bladder of low capacity with a residual urine is a common condition in old age. Continence is previously maintained in the presence of considerable functional impairment. The incontinent state is precipitated by a further factor or stress such as a change of environment, physical or mental disease. Some causes of incontinence may be simply summarized in the incontinence flow chart (Fig. 12).

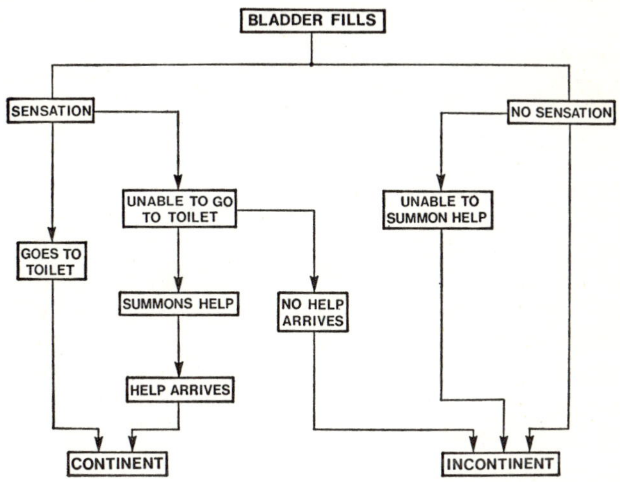

FIG. 12. An incontinence flow-chart.

Management

As has been mentioned before, investigations and treatment will be far more effective if carried out in an atmosphere where incontinence is treated as a challenge to be overcome, and not as something to be borne and accepted. By keeping the patients alert and stimulated with various interests, their outlook may be broadened and the incidence of incontinence reduced.

Incontinence may be prevented if the nursing staff adopt a positive approach to the situation and exercise tolerance. The patient's dignity must be maintained, also his self-respect and individuality. The nurse must also remember the importance of privacy to the patient and remember to draw the curtains and always shut the door of the lavatory, so that the patient is not left exposed for all who are passing to see. It is essential that the nurse remembers to leave the patient for only a short period of time as he may become cold and uncomfortable. Pants should be worn by the patient whenever possible. There should be easy access to the lavatory or commode; the lavatories should be clearly marked or coloured and all new patients shown where they are situated.

A pattern of incontinence should be established and this may be done with the aid of an incontinence chart (Fig. 13). This task should be allocated each day to a particular nurse, who should understand its tremendous importance, and also that it is a very necessary though time-consuming job. The patient should be taken to the lavatory or commode or offered a urinal every 2 hours, and the nurse should record on the chart whether the patient is wet or dry, and whether or not he passes urine or faeces. After a few days a pattern of incontinence should evolve which will assist in planning further investigation and treatment. It may be necessary to measure the residual urine, as inefficient micturition and incomplete emptying of the bladder are increasingly common in old age.

A gynaecological examination is usually carried out by the doctor on all incontinent female patients to eliminate the possibility of a cystocele, uterine prolapse or abnormality of the pelvic floor. The male patient will have a rectal examination to detect the presence of an enlarged prostate gland and at the same time a bimanual examination may be carried out. Routine investigations should include measurement of blood urea, renal function tests, intravenous pyelogram where necessary and cystometry. Cystometric studies have improved

INCONTINENCE CHART	UNIT No.	
	SURNAME (Block letters)	Mr Mrs Miss
Ward	FIRST NAMES	

Date														
TIME	Commode or Bed Pan given by	U.F. or Dry	Commode or Bed Pan given by	U.F. or Dry	Commode or Bed Pan given by	U.F. or Dry	Commode or Bed Pan given by	U.F. or Dry	Commode or Bed Pan given by	U.F. or Dry	Commode or Bed Pan given by	U.F. or Dry	Commode or Bed Pan given by	U.F. or Dry
a.m. 8														
10														
12														
p.m. 2														
4														
6														
8														
10														
12														
a.m. 2														
4														
6														

FIG. 13. An incontinence chart.

understanding of bladder functioning. The cystometer determines both the capacity and function of the urinary bladder. A fluid balance chart should be kept initially when possible, to record not only an adequate intake of fluid, but also the output of urine.

If the incontinence is due to cerebral arteriosclerosis, a cerebrovascular accident or immobility, the patient may benefit from a period of habit training. This again must be carried out in a tranquil atmosphere and the patient allotted to a particular nurse for the day. The patient should be encouraged to go to the lavatory every 1–2 hours initially and the time span gradually increased as training progresses with the resumption of continence, and the improvement noted on the incontinence chart. This regimen should be continued at night and the importance explained to the night staff.

All ambulant patients should be allowed and assisted to go to the lavatory, and the less ambulant aided by the Sanichair. For those who are not able to help themselves, a commode or urinal may be used, and only on very rare occasions as a last resort, the bedpan. If used regularly, the bedpan makes difficulties later for the patient who will not have such facilities when he is discharged home or to residential accommodation. Patients balanced precariously on the bedpan in an uncomfortable position in bed, agitated at the thought of missing the pan and wetting the bed, are unlikely to be able to pass urine satisfactorily.

Nocturnal Incontinence

Some patients are troubled by nocturnal incontinence alone and again this must also be dealt with positively and optimistically, as it is not only demoralizing for them, but may make it difficult for their relations to have them home or for them to be accepted for residential accommodation. In order to help them overcome this problem, the patients should be encouraged to drink well during the day, and fluids should be restricted after 5 p.m. in the evening. This should be explained to the patient and the staff so that confusion and misunderstanding does not arise.

Many elderly people are accustomed to having a bucket or chamber pot under the bed at home, and find the journey to the ward lavatory too long and difficult at night. However, this can easily be remedied by leaving a commode near the bed so that they can get in and out to this at their convenience. Some may need to be awakened and helped to the commode at regular intervals during the night, but this does not tend to disturb them unduly. Night sedation should be used with care, as many patients complain that they lose control at night if they have a hypnotic drug. In fact some patients benefit from an amphetamine so that they sleep lightly and wake automatically when they need to micturate.

Use of Drugs

There are some drugs which have a direct effect on incontinence and should be used with care. Diuretics frequently tip the balance into incontinence in a previously continent patient, and it will be very difficult to control the incontinence if it is necessary for the patient to continue with the diuretic. A large proportion of the elderly are given diuretics to control incipient congestive cardiac failure; some may need a mild and gentle action, some need a stronger diuretic in larger doses.

Cetiprin (emepronium bromide) and Urispas (flavoxate hydrochloride) may be used to help control incontinence. These drugs have an antichlolinergic effect increasing the bladder capacity by blocking the transmission of nervous impulses somewhere within the sacral reflex arc. Urispas is supplied as 100 mg tablets and the dosage is up to 2 tablets 3 times daily. Cetiprin is supplied as 50 mg and 100 mg tablets and the dosage is up to 200 mg three times daily and 400 mg at night. Myotonine (bethanechol chloride) may be used in cases of urinary retention and bladder dysfunction. Disipidin snuff containing antidiuretic hormone can sometimes be used at night for those with nocturnal incontinence.

Catheterization

Some patients with an atonic bladder benefit either from a permanent indwelling catheter or from a short-term catheter released 4-hourly during the day in order to improve the muscle tone of the bladder.

Technique Catheterization must be carried out with great care and aseptically, in order not to introduce infection into the bladder either from the catheter or the external genitalia. The nurse should explain carefully the procedure to the patient before she starts, giving the reasons for the necessity of an indwelling catheter. If possible the nurse should bath the patient before she begins and the patient should be in a clean bed in the recumbent position with the knees flexed, covered by a blanket. It is normally best to have another nurse present to reassure the patient, and help maintain the correct position, as many elderly people find it uncomfortable and tiring.

Female catheterization Requirements for female catheterization are:

Prepared sterile catheter of suitable size and type according to the requirements of the patient
2 sterile dressing forceps or sterile gloves
Pair of sterile scissors

Container for used instruments
Disposable bag for dirty dressings
Bowl of lotion for swabbing (Savlon or Hibitane 1/100)
Sterile swabs and 3 sterile towels
Large receiver for urine
Good lighting
If the catheter is self-retaining, syringe, and sterile water to inflate the balloon
Urine drainage bag or spigot

The nurse opens her sterile containers, prepares the lotion and washes her hands. She places the towels over both legs and the abdomen. Using swabs soaked in an acceptable antiseptic solution, she swabs first the external genitalia, beginning with the labia majora, then the labia minora and the urethral orifice. Each swab is used once in a downwards direction, and as the labia are cleaned, they are held apart by the free hand. Eventually the urethra should be clearly seen, and the catheter inserted by the nurse either wearing sterile gloves or using a pair of sterile dissecting forceps, the end of the catheter being kept in the sterile receiver. It must not be allowed to touch the surrounding skin, as this would be a potential source of infection. The residual urine may then be drained and the catheter removed. If the catheter is self-retaining, the bulb should be blown up with the appropriate amount of sterile water using a sterile syringe; it is then attached to a drainage bag or spigotted, a sterile specimen of urine having been collected to send to the laboratory.

If the purpose of the catheter is to retrain the bladder muscle, it may be necessary to release the catheter 2–4-hourly depending on the patient's comfort and bladder capacity. When this is done a sterile spigot must be used each time, the urine drained into a sterile container and the whole procedure carried out aseptically. Under certain circumstances the catheter may be clamped and released intermittently to drain into a urine bag.

Male catheterization Male catheterization is generally carried out only by an experienced male nurse or doctor. Requirements for male catheterization are:

Prepacked catheters of the required type
Lubricant—sterile glycerine, liquid paraffin or KY jelly
Sterile gloves
2 pairs of dissecting forceps
Container for used instruments
Disposable bag for dirty dressings
1 pair sterile scissors
Sterile towels and swabs
Bowl of lotion for swabbing (Savlon or Hibitane 1/100)
If catheter is self-retaining, syringe and sterile water to inflate the bulb
Urine drainage bag or spigot
Good lighting

The patient is prepared as described for female catheterization and the nurse gets ready the dressing pack and lotion before washing his hands and putting on a pair of sterile gloves. The towels are placed, so as to prepare a large sterile area leaving the patient as little exposed as possible. The meatus and prepuce are carefully cleansed, and the catheter is lubricated and passed without force until urine is obtained.

If the catheter is withdrawn after the bladder is emptied, it should be removed gradually and the meatus swabbed. If the catheter is to be left in position, it may be fixed by the use of tape, or one of the self-retaining variety of catheter used.

Management Drainage bags should be changed aseptically, and should be changed, not emptied, preferably once a day, or more often if the amount of urine passed is large.

Patients who are ambulant should be fitted with a leg bag (Fig. 14) which is unobtrusive, being attached to the leg under a man's trousers or a woman's stocking. The bag has a one-

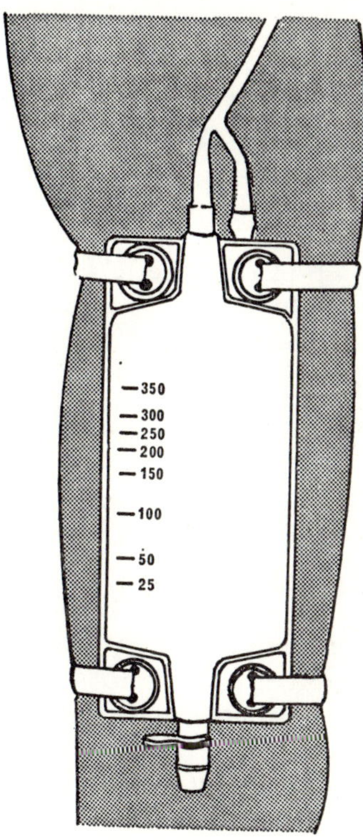

FIG. 14. A leg drainage bag.

way valve to prevent the urine leaking back into the catheter. There is nothing more degrading or unpleasant for the patient or his companions than to have to sit with a urine bag dangling from a walking frame or chair for all to see. Infection and blockage of the catheter may be prevented by inserting a solution of neomycin 0·2% with 2 ampoules of Elase for 30 minutes into the catheter and then washing it out with 2 litres of normal saline whenever the catheter is changed.

Catheters should be changed routinely every 2–3 weeks, but there are now Silastic catheters which do not decompose within the bladder, and necessitate changing less frequently; these are very useful for long-term catheterization.

Indications There are situations when a catheter is clearly indicated:

1. When a patient is unable to go home or to an old people's home purely because he or she is incontinent.
2. When there is a pressure sore present which requires active treatment.
3. When the incontinence increases the risk of the development of a pressure sore.

Case history An elderly lady was admitted from an old people's home with a history of urinary incontinence for 2 years. She constantly wet the bed at night and occasionally the chair where she was sitting, and had become very unpopular with other residents because of the constant unpleasant odour.

Investigations revealed that she had a urinary tract infection which was treated with the appropriate antibiotic, and also that she had an atonic bladder with a residual urine of 1000 ml. A self-retaining catheter was inserted, spigotted and released 4-hourly, for 2 weeks, in an effort to retrain the bladder muscle. The catheter was then removed and the patient taken to the lavatory 2-hourly. The first day passed successfully, but day by day the situation deteriorated, and after 5 days and many disasters her residual urine was 800 ml. It was decided that the best solution was to leave an indwelling catheter in situ, attached to a leg bag during the day, and an ordinary drainage bag at night. The old lady was very happy, as she dreaded the incontinent episodes and learnt to change and empty her own bag. The home was happy to accept her with the catheter, and it was arranged that the home nurse would change it at regular intervals.

Aids for Incontinence

There are various appliances for the incontinent patient for whom catheterization may not be practical or necessary.

For the male incontinent patient *Penile clamps* These are not often used as their siting must be exact so as to be effective without causing oedema of the penis.

Rubber urinals These consist of a suspensory belt with a rubber sheath fitting over the penis, which is attached to a leg bag. The rubber sheath sometimes irritates the surrounding skin; however, the modern pubic pressure urinals have overcome this problem by making a short inner sleeve which fits round the pubis and base of the penis, and the outer condom remains loose.

Portex disposable urine bags These can be attached to the scrotum by a drawstring. They are strong and light, allowing freedom of movement and causing minimal irritation.

Dribbler bags These are a recent introduction from Scandinavia, and consist basically of a plastic bag, of which there are two designs—the first is a plain bag and the second has a non-return valve for extra confidence. They are attached by a draw-string and are very simple and easy to manage.

For the female incontinent patient Aids for females are less efficient as some leakage of urine on to the skin is bound to occur.

Incontinence pants A variety of designs are available which can be worn in conjunction with an absorbent pad which may need to be changed at regular intervals.

Polyweb incontinence pads (Fig. 15) These are manufactured

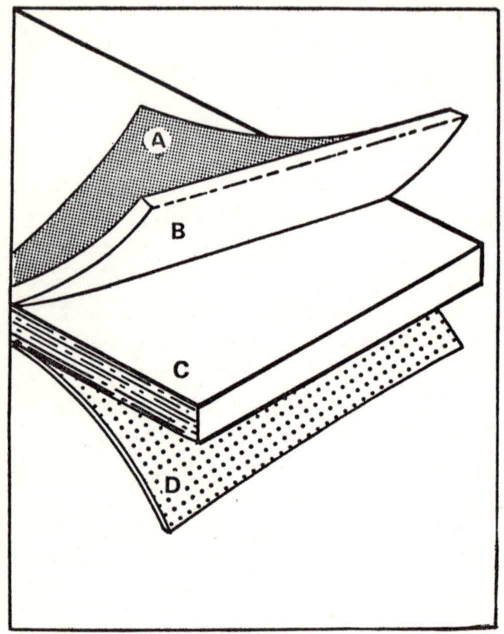

FIG. 15. A Polyweb incontinence pad. A, Polyweb facing material. B, White absorbent fleece. C, Absorbent cellulose wadding. D, Non-slip polythene backing.

by Smith and Nephew and are a great asset in saving laundry. They can absorb a large quantity of urine, and the plastic net webbing will keep the patient dry, and help to reduce bed-sores and rashes. They consist of four layers—the Polyweb facing, white absorbent fleece which enables fluid to pass to the next layer, thick cellulose wadding which absorbs much fluid, and non-slip polythene backing which keeps the linen dry and prevents the pad coming out of place. They are available in 3 sizes.

The nurse must remember that urinary incontinence must be viewed objectively and sympathetically, and during the investigations and subsequent management, the patients must always be treated with the utmost respect and courtesy, thus retaining their dignity and self-respect. Patience on the part of both patient and nurse combined with modern methods and aids can do a great deal to reduce incontinence and alleviate the patient's discomfort and distress.

Faecal Incontinence

Cause Faecal incontinence is far less common than urinary incontinence and the most usual cause is faecal impaction. Other causes are diarrhoea caused by carcinoma of the colon, proctitis, colitis and non-specific diarrhoea resulting from poor diet. Rectal prolapse and haemorrhoids occur especially in the elderly grand multipara due to weakness or incompetence of the pelvic floor.

The elderly frequently become obsessed with their bowels and are distressed if they have not passed one loose motion every day. As a result they tend to take various favourite purgatives. This may have been their practice for some years, with the result that the colon no longer reacts to stimulation and becomes over-distended. Eventually constant stretching of the rectum and pelvic colon produces weakness and lack of tone of the muscular wall. The bulk of faecal mass tends to be small and hard thus failing to stimulate reflex action in the rectum, which anyway is frequently diminished in later life.

Faecal impaction is caused by constipation in a person confined to bed, dehydration from diminished fluid intake, the use of high residue food substances or bulk laxatives and analgesics such as codeine. The large bowel becomes overloaded and the faecal mass becomes dry and hard, causing loss of sphincter control. Eventually the hard faeces in the rectum act as an irritant to the mucosal lining and the mucous secreted dissolves some of the faecal mass causing a little liquid stool to be excreted in the form of spurious diarrhoea.

Signs and symptoms Faecal impaction is usually suspected from the soiling of the patient's underwear or drawsheet and the typical stale offensive smell of faecal matter. It is diagnosed by abdominal examination, indentation of the faecal masses on rectal examination and plain X-ray of the abdomen, particularly for high impaction.

Treatment The treatment is to soften the stool with Dioctyl or Dorbanex. These are combinations of a wetting agent and a mild peristaltic stimulant which, given at night, prevent further impaction. The patient should then begin daily enemas until the result of the enema is the return of fluid free from faecal matter. Initially it may be necessary to do a digital removal of the stool if it is very hard, but this should only be undertaken by an experienced nurse or doctor.

A few patients are unable to tolerate an enema, and then 4 or 5 glycerine suppositories may be inserted by the nurse. Once the bowel is empty, constipation should be prevented by giving a mild aperient or stool softener, and glycerine suppositories. Faulty dietary habits causing malnutrition, lack of vitamins and roughage should be corrected. Fluid intake should be encouraged. Faulty toilet habits and impaired mental awareness may be improved with a period of training. Very occasionally faecal impaction causes subacute intestinal obstruction, and the patient with a ball of faeces as large as a melon in the caecal region has been known to undergo a laparotomy to relieve the obstruction.

Complications Overloading of the sigmoid colon and rectum in impaction may obstruct the bladder and impair control perhaps leading to retention with overflow and urinary incontinence.

Diverticulosis and diverticulitis may be caused and aggravated by constipation and impaction. Small diverticula are found in 5–10% of persons over middle age, most commonly in the pelvic colon. Diverticulosis is symptomless. If the openings in the diverticulae become narrow, faecal material may stagnate in the pouches and infection occurs, giving rise to symptoms and an acute form of the disease known as diverticulitis with all its complications.

Inflammatory changes lead to thickening of the affected area of the colon which may be adherent to the surrounding structures causing fistulae, perforation or haemorrhage. The disease may flare up for periods over many years causing abdominal pain, generally left-sided and associated with defaecation. Occasionally a mass is felt in the left iliac fossa and may be confused with a carcinoma. Diagnosis is made by sigmoidoscopy and barium enema. Treatment is to give a well-balanced diet that is non-irritating and yet prevents constipation occurring. Bulk-producing aperients such as Isogel may be used.

Non-specific diarrhoea will be improved by giving a well balanced diet and regular doses of kaolin. Proctitis and colitis may be treated with an anti-inflammatory drug or a bulk maker. Occasionally it may be necessary to give a short course of oral steroids or a retention enema containing steroids.

Rectal prolapse may occur, causing loss of sphincter control and incontinence. There is weakness of the muscles of the pelvic floor as the result of chronic constipation and the rectal wall protrudes through the anus. Surgical treatment may be necessary with the insertion of a ring or tantalum wire round the anus. Great care must be exercised to ensure that faecal impaction does not follow surgery.

Neuromuscular incoordination of the anal sphincter has been successfully treated by a battery-operated pulsator. Severe cerebral damage due to a cerebrovascular accident or cerebral arteriosclerosis will produce lack of cortical control leading to faecal incontinence, but the patient may respond to the regular use of suppositories or enemas.

Method of giving an enema A fully comprehensive explanation must be given to the patient by the nurse before the procedure is begun. The windows are closed and the patient laid on the bed on his left side with his knees drawn up, the bed having been well protected with a disposable draw sheet and incontinence pads. A commode should be placed near the bedside. The nurse will prepare a tray containing:

Enema tubing and funnel
Rectal tube
Enema solution warmed to 38°C
Tissues
Fresh-aire aerosol
Lubricant
Pair of disposable gloves
Disposal bag for receipt of the used rectal tube

The rectal tube is attached to the tubing and funnel and the nurse runs some enema solution through the apparatus to displace any air present. The lubricated rectal tube is inserted into the rectum and gently guided as far as it will go. The enema solution is slowly run in until the patient feels he can hold no more. He is then seated upon the commode and evacuation of the enema will take place. It may take some

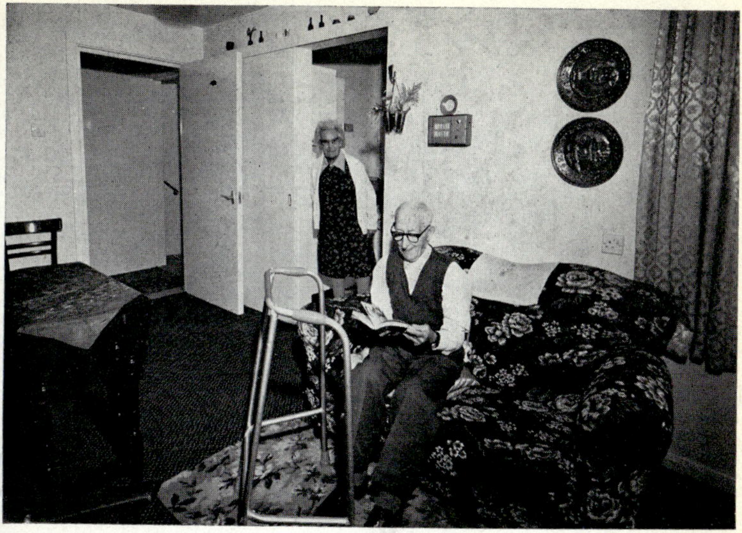

PLATE I. A warden controlled flat.

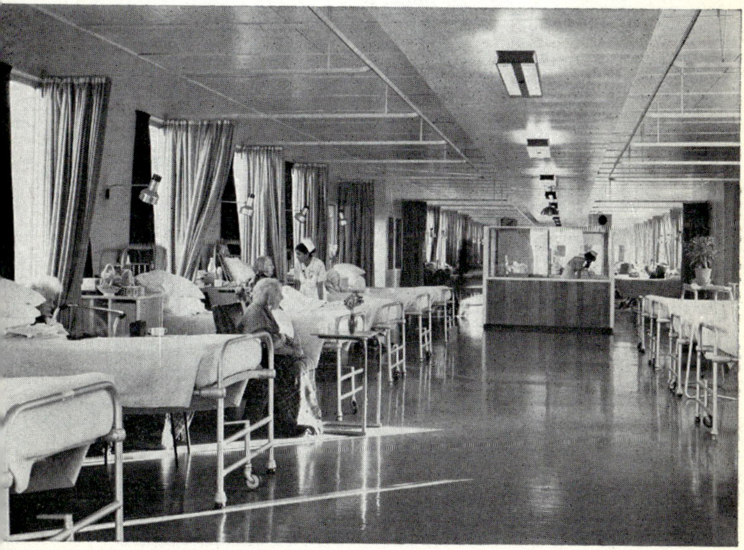

PLATE II. An assessment and rehabilitation ward.

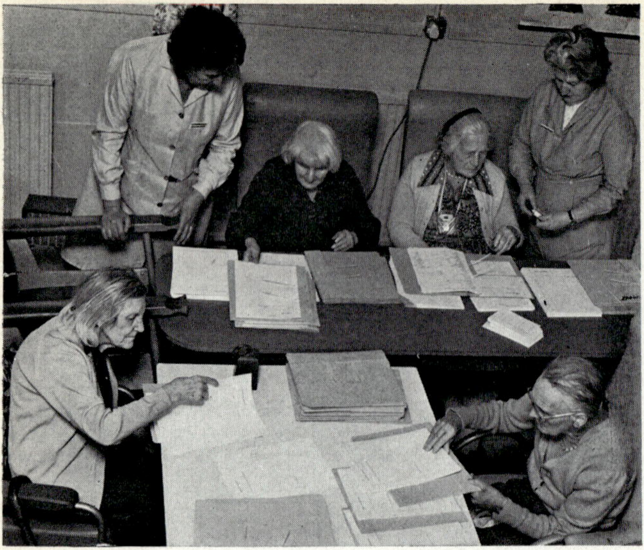

PLATE III. Work in the day hospital.

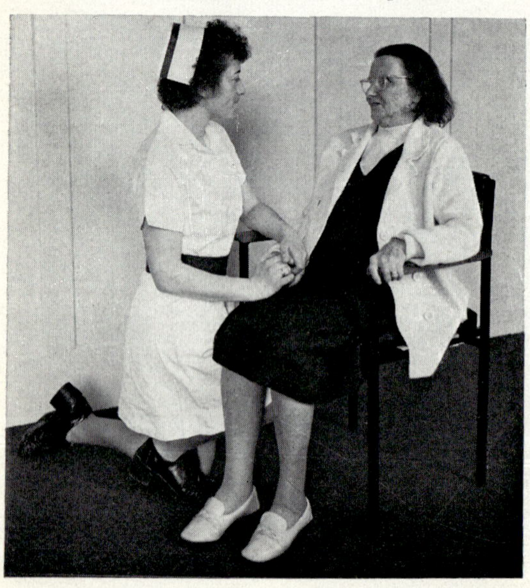

PLATE IV. The correct way to address an elderly patient.

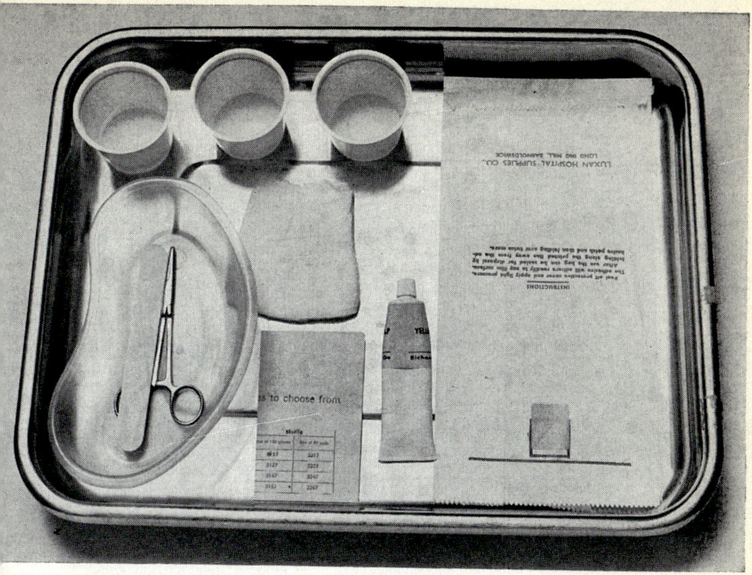

PLATE V. An oral tray.

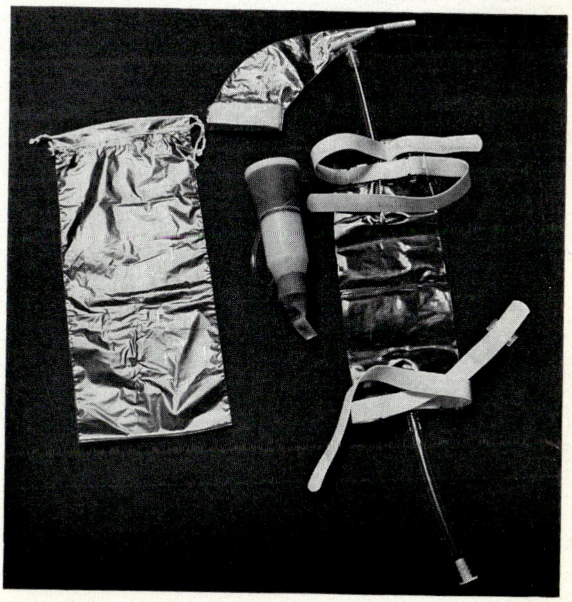

PLATE VI. A male urinal, non-spill bag and a Portex disposable urine bag.

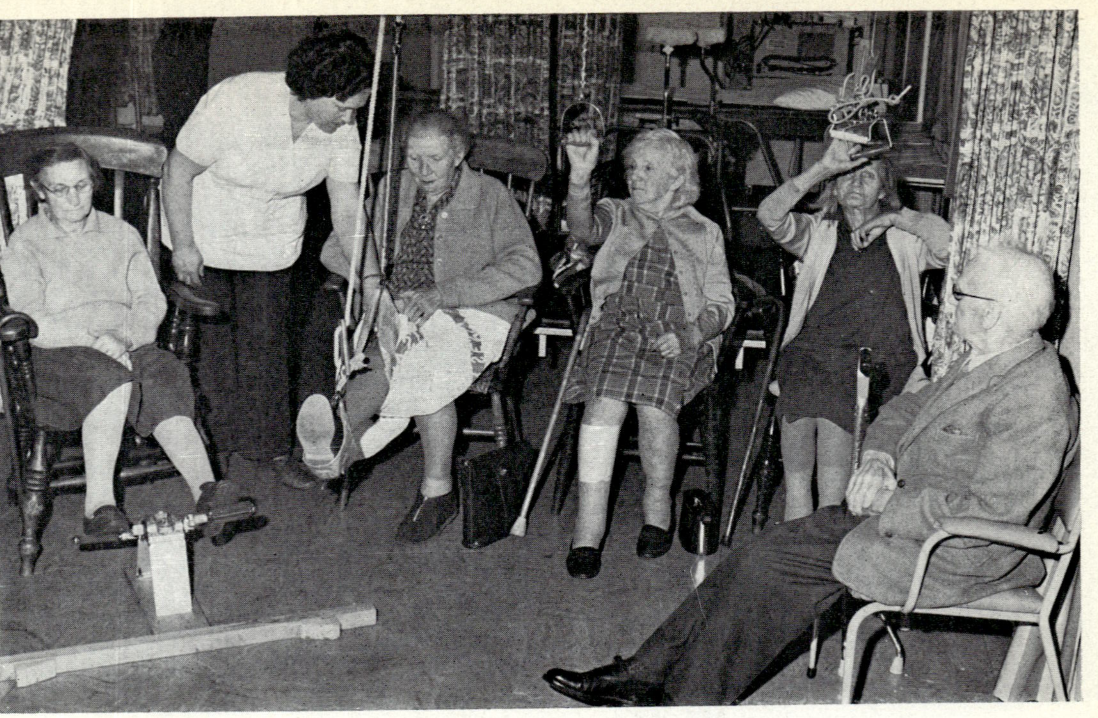

PLATE VII. Group physiotherapy.

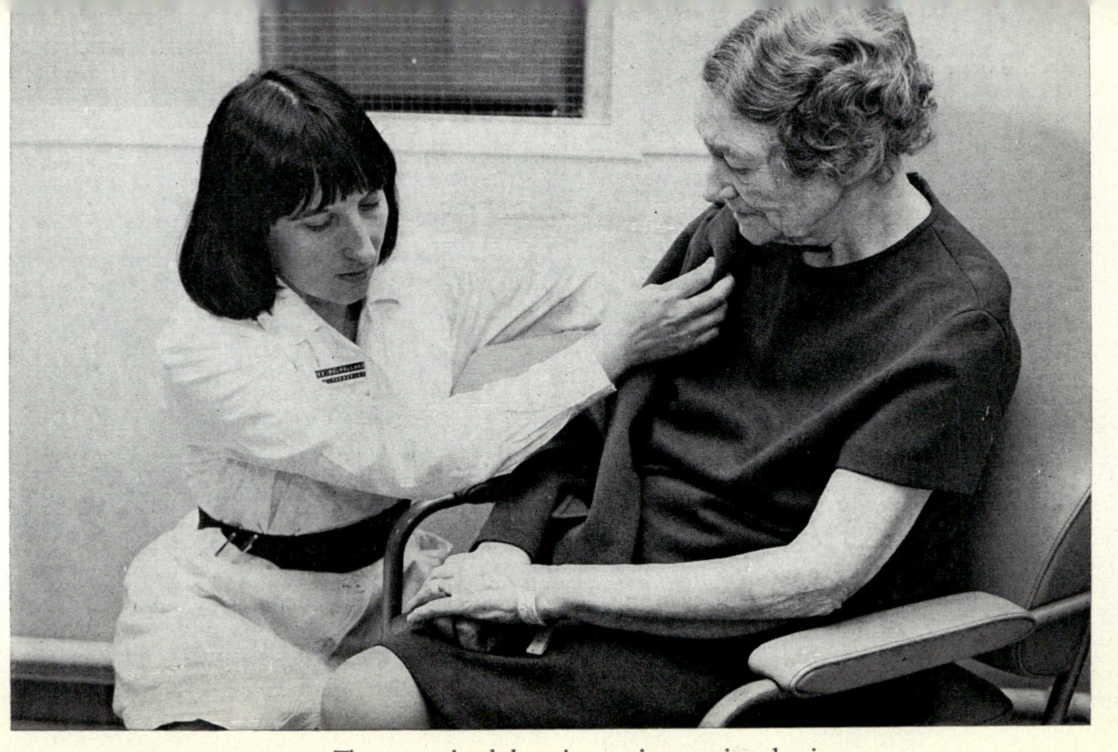

PLATE VIII. The occupational therapist assessing a patient dressing.

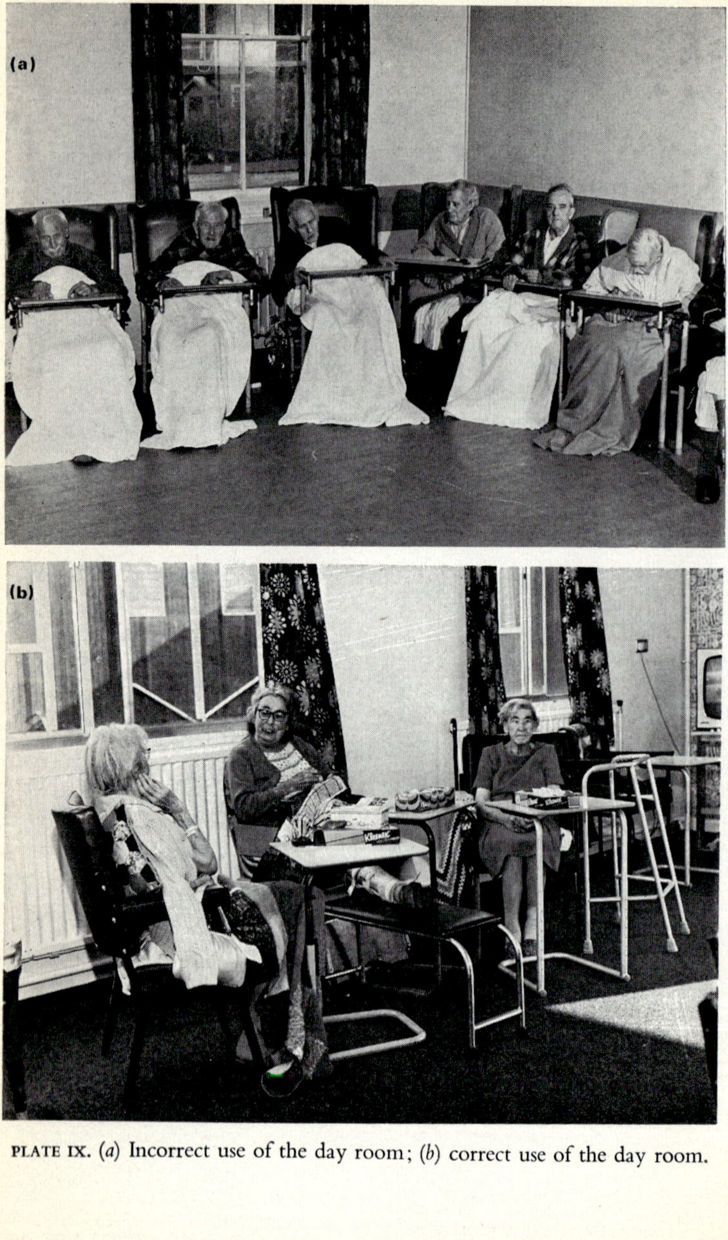

(a)

(b)

PLATE IX. (*a*) Incorrect use of the day room; (*b*) correct use of the day room.

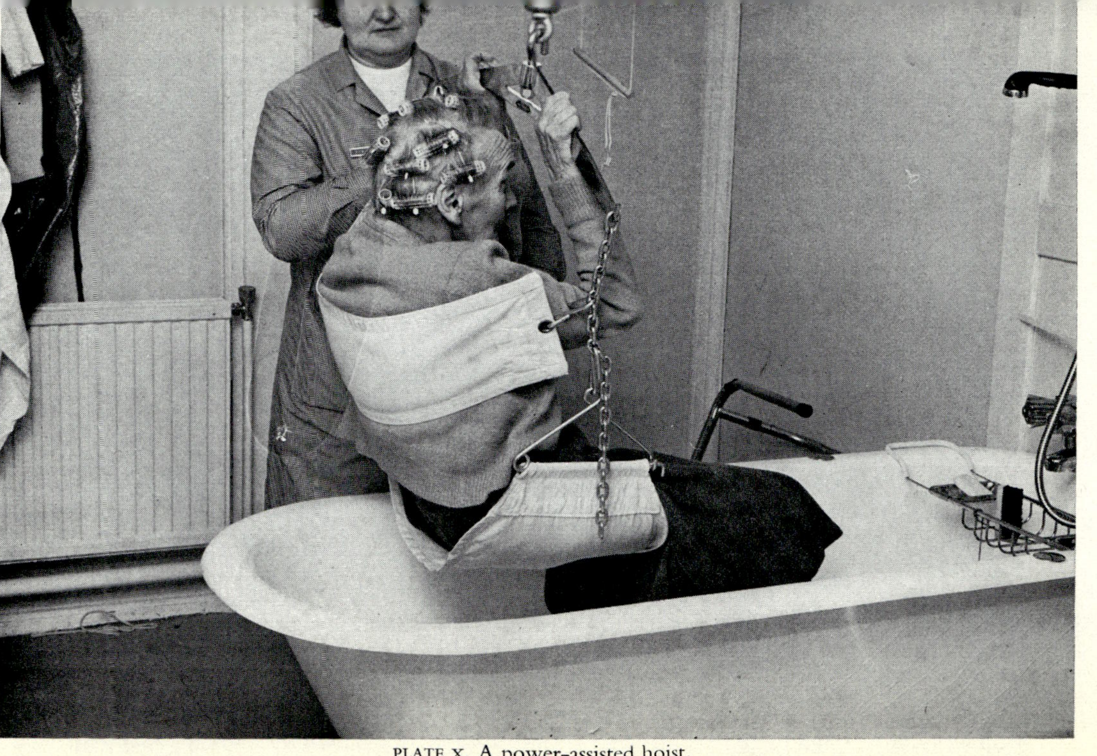

PLATE X. A power-assisted hoist.

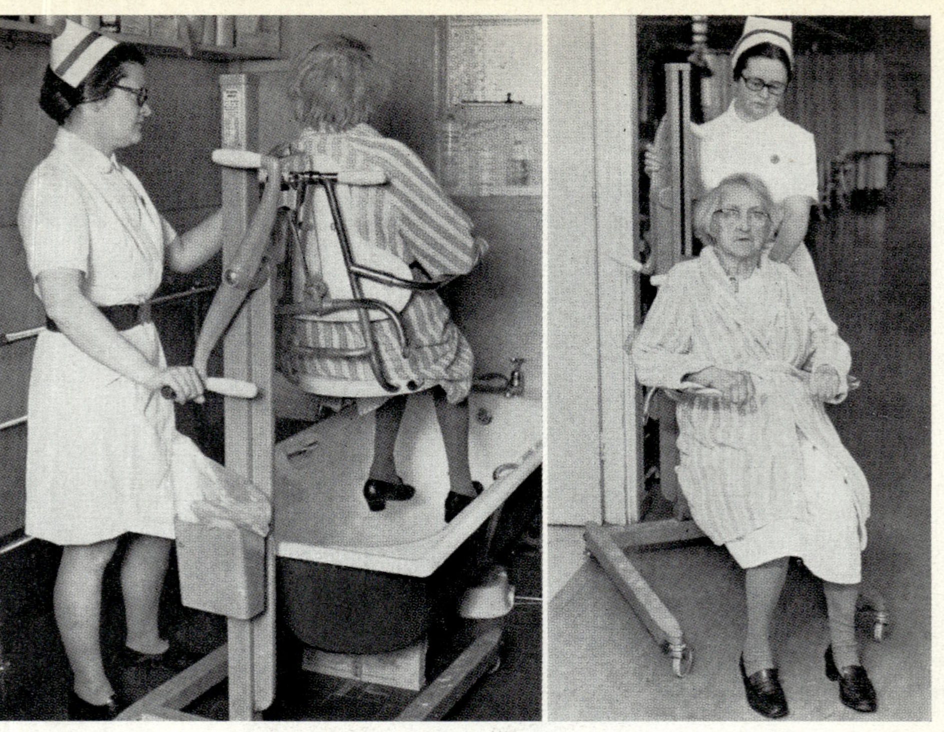

PLATE XI. The Ambulift.

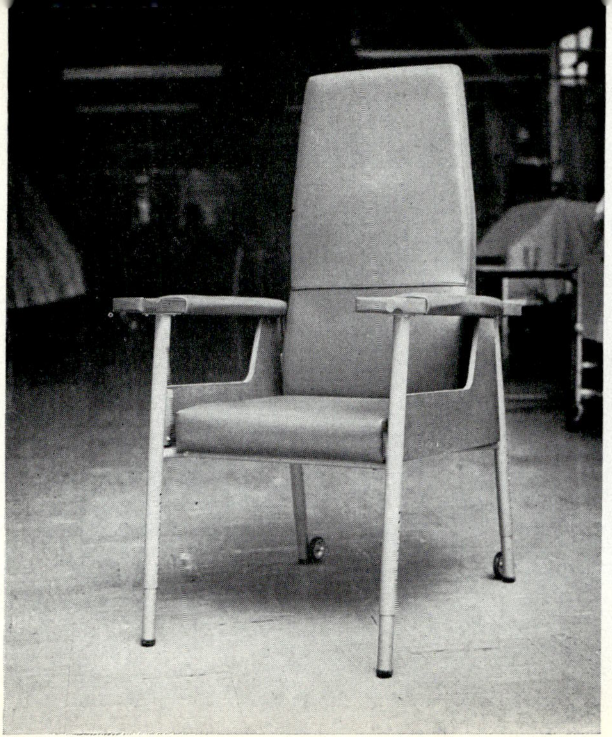

PLATE XII. The Easy-to-Rise Chair.

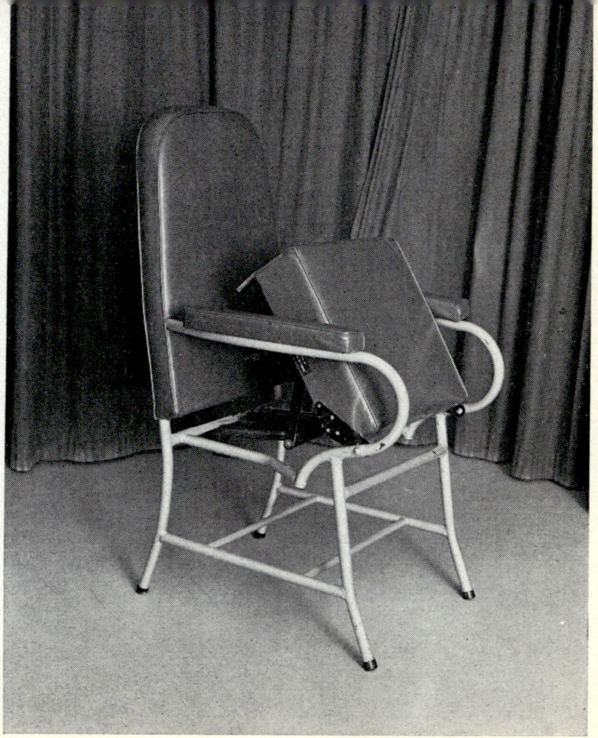

PLATE XIII. The Self-Lift Chair.

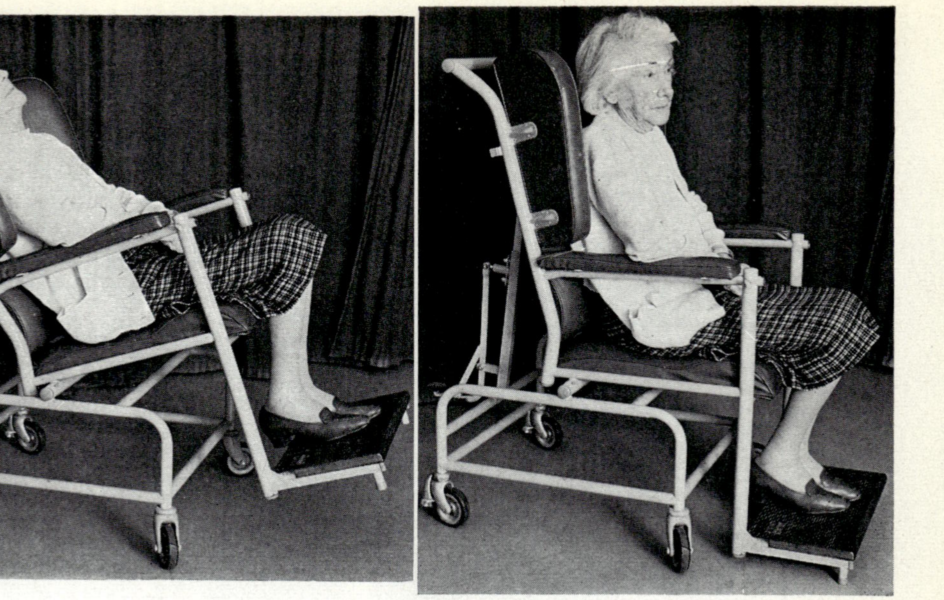

PLATE XIV. The Buxton Chair.

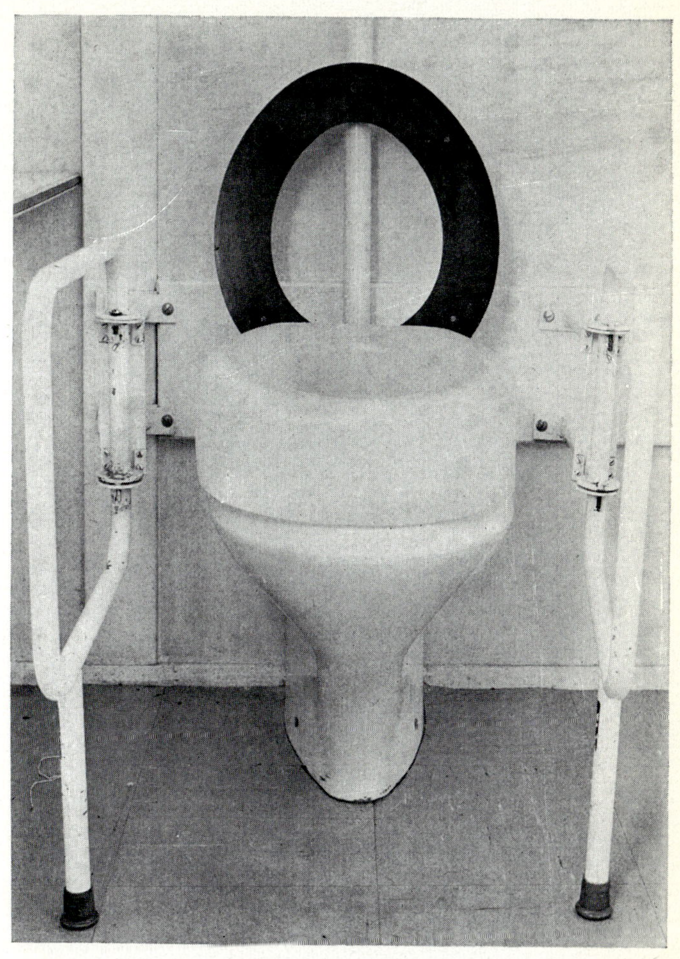

PLATE XV. Lavatory seat and aids.

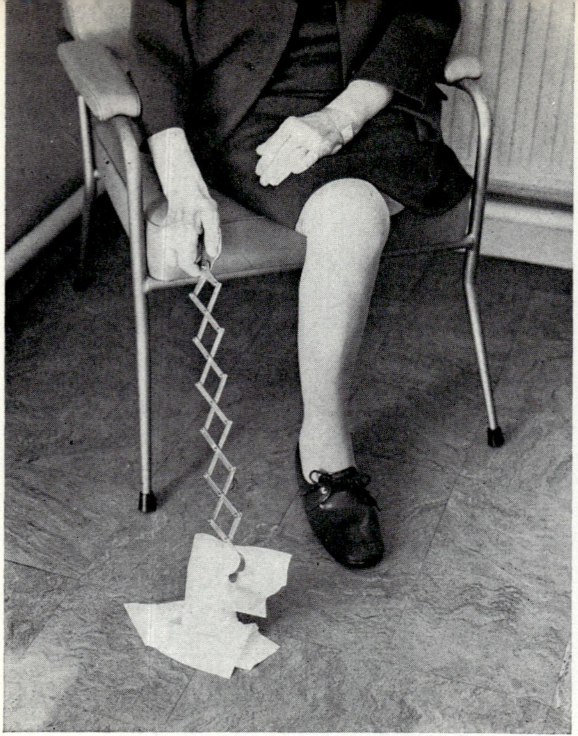

PLATE XVI. Lazy tongs.

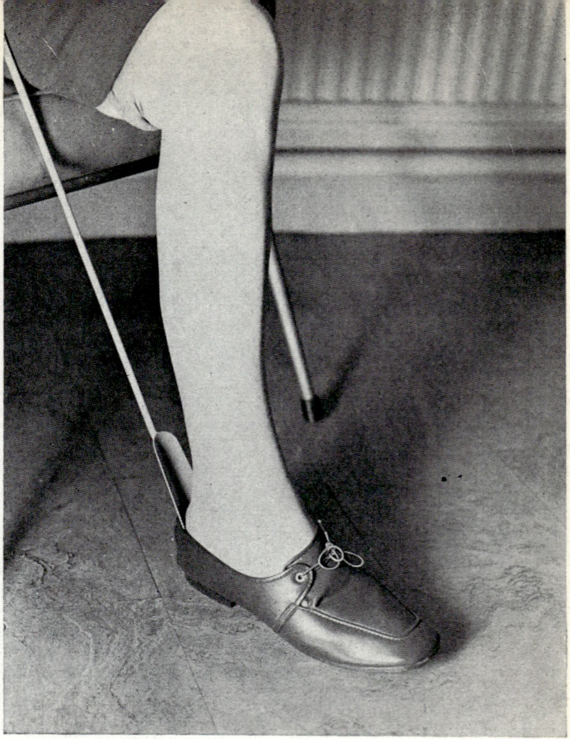

PLATE XVII. Long-handled shoehorn and elastic shoelaces.

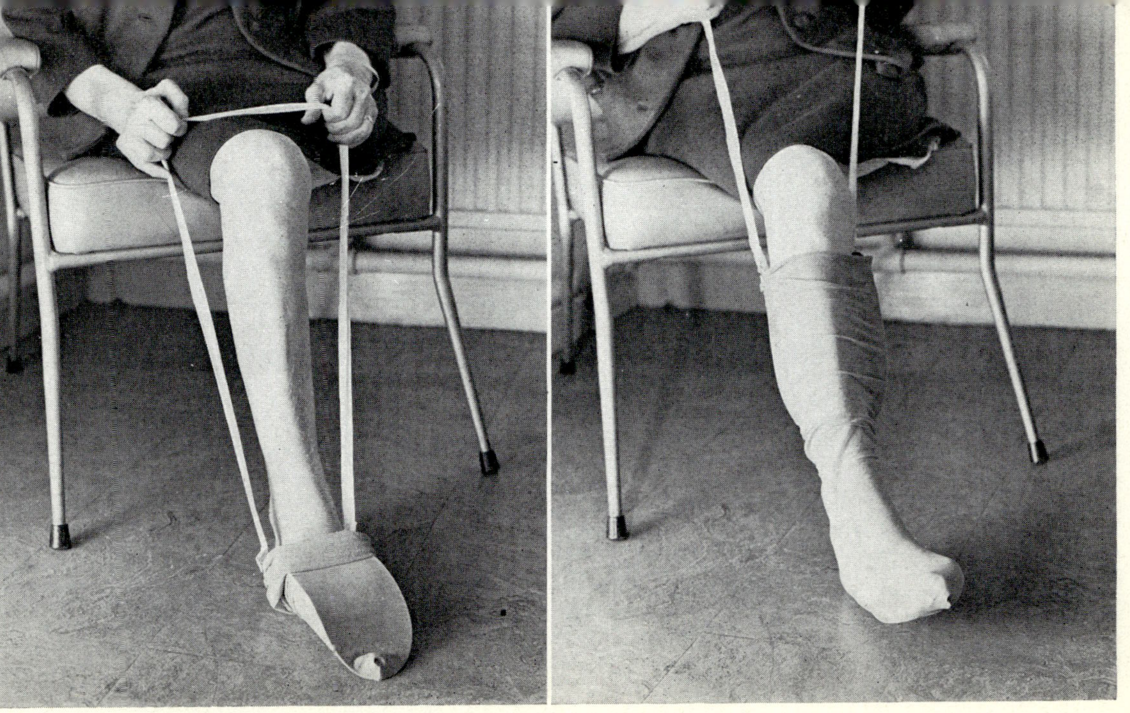

PLATE XVIII. Stocking gutter.

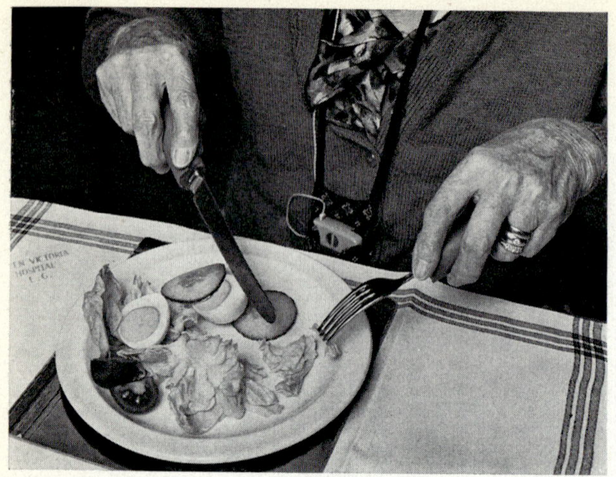

PLATE XIX. Cutlery handles covered with Rubazote sponge.

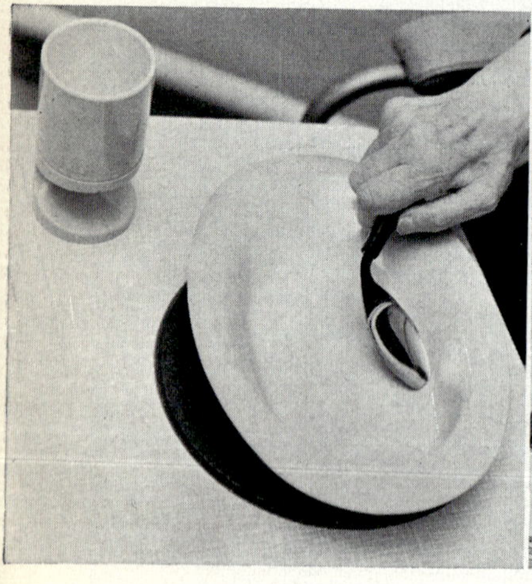

PLATE XX. The Manoy range of crockery and cutlery.

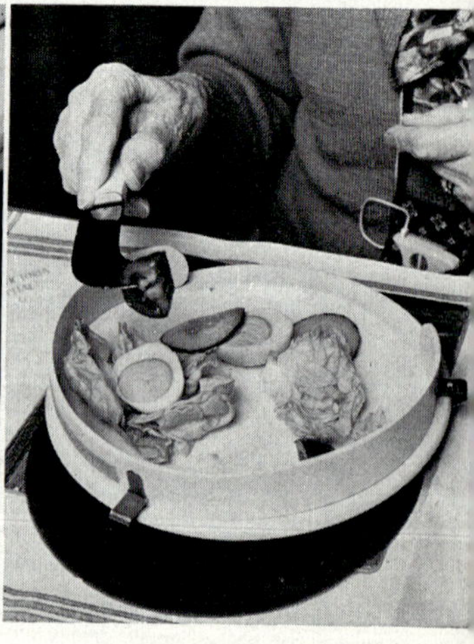

PLATE XXI. Nelson knife, non-slip mat and plastic bunker.

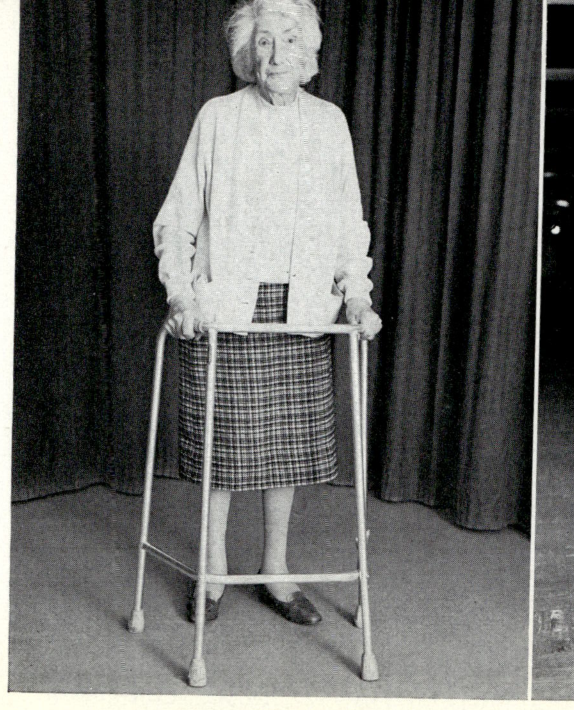

PLATE XXII. Walking frame.

PLATE XXIII. Rollator.

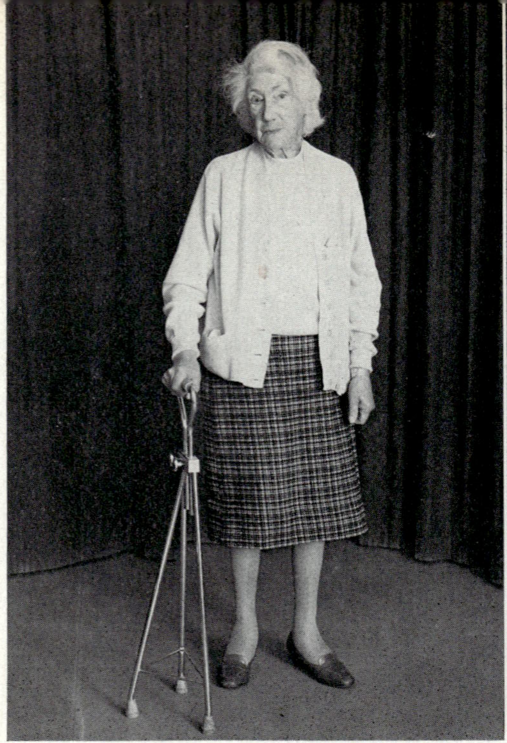

PLATE XXIV. Tripod.

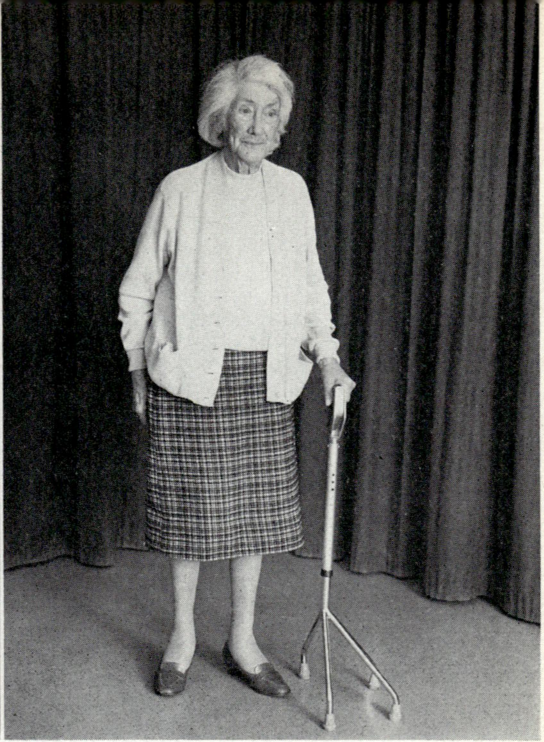

PLATE XXV. Quadriped.

considerable time and the patient should be left in a comfortable position, the nurse ensuring that he is quite warm. When the procedure is completed, the patient usually appreciates a warm bath. The most commonly used and apparently most effective enema is the enema saponis. This is made up with a small lump of enema soap about the size of a walnut, dissolved in 1 litre of water and given at a temperature of 37·8°C (100°F). The elderly patient usually tolerates 250–500 ml.

The disposable sodium phosphate enema, previously warmed in a bowl of hot water, may be given, but is less effective. A rectal tube needs to be connected to the end of the tube, so that it can be inserted fairly high up in the rectum.

Gentle and more lubricating is the glycerine enema; 60 ml of glycerine are added to 200 ml of warm water, and the enema is run in slowly and retained for 20–30 minutes.

In very severe cases of impaction, when the patient is fit, an olive oil retention enema may be given to be retained overnight. 100–250 ml of warm olive oil are slowly run into the rectum and the bed is tipped on blocks for the night. This is followed by an enema saponis the next morning.

The enemas should be given with the patient lying on his left side with the knees drawn up if possible. The nurse should protect the bed with a disposable drawsheet and incontinence pads and have a commode near at hand. The nurse should explain the procedure clearly to the patient before she starts, reassure him and make sure that he is kept warm.

In conclusion it must be said that urinary incontinence is on the whole controllable and faecal incontinence preventable. The success of the treatment will depend very largely upon the atmosphere within the ward and the optimistic attitude of the staff.

6 Pressure Sores and their Prevention

Much of the nurse's time within the geriatric unit is concerned with the prevention of the formation of pressure sores, and also with the treatment of these sores when they are present. Some 12·5 % of geriatric patients admitted to hospital have pressure sores and their presence increases the amount of nursing needed by 50 %. A sore can form very rapidly within a day and takes months to heal, therefore the treatment and prevention are extremely important and deserve much consideration. The onus for this falls mainly on the nursing staff with help and advice from the medical staff and physiotherapists.

Development of pressure sores interferes considerably with the patient's rehabilitation and may be a contributory cause of death. A survey done by Exton-Smith, Maclaren and Norton in 1964 showed that the mortality rate was five times as great in those who developed sores and the length of stay in hospital was much longer, although it must be remembered that those who had pressure sores were generally more debilitated than those who did not. Pressure sores occurring in hospital are still regarded as a sign of bad nursing with shame and guilt by the nursing staff. However, sores can develop despite an excellent standard of care and the administration of all the necessary precautions by the staff. Their task can be aided, and they can be guided in this difficult field by the devising of a simple scoring system, whereby the patient's mental and physical condition is assessed (Fig. 16). A high score will reveal a fairly able, alert and ambulant patient, and a low score, a debilitated, confused incontinent patient who is greatly at risk. This system will also identify those borderline

.... HOSPITAL PRESSURE SORE RISK AND PROGRESS CHART Ward	UNIT No. SURNAME (block letters) Mr./Mrs./Miss FIRST NAMES AGE

Scoring System. Total score of 14 or below equals 'At Risk'

A. Physical State	Good 4	Fair 3	Poor 2	V. Bad 1
B. Mental State	Good 4	Confused 3	Apathetic 2	Stuperous 1
C. Activity	Ambulant 4	Walk/Help 3	Chairfast 2	Bedfast 1
D. Mobility	Full 4	Sl. Limited 3	V. Limited 2	Immobile 1
E. Incontinence	None 4	Occasional 3	Usual/Ur. 2	Double 1

Date	A	B	C	D	E	Total	Remarks
A81SO							

FIG. 16. A pressure sore 'at risk' chart.

cases who need constant attention. The system should be reviewed weekly to assess those who deteriorate and those who improve. The patients can then be grouped into those needing intensive care, those requiring intermediate care and those who require only supervision, and the nurses' work allocated accordingly. In some units the patients' care is indicated by colour coding over the bed, in others the nursing care required is recorded in the Kardex. It is essential that all the nursing staff are aware of those at risk and that nurses are allocated specific patients to care for, so that a high standard of care can be maintained day and night. This is one of the reasons for the high ratio of nursing staff to patients referred to in Chapter 2.

Types of Sore

The common sites of sores when the patient is recumbent (Fig. 17) are shoulders, sacrum, elbows and heels. In the severely debilitated patient, sores can also develop on the ears and the back of the head.

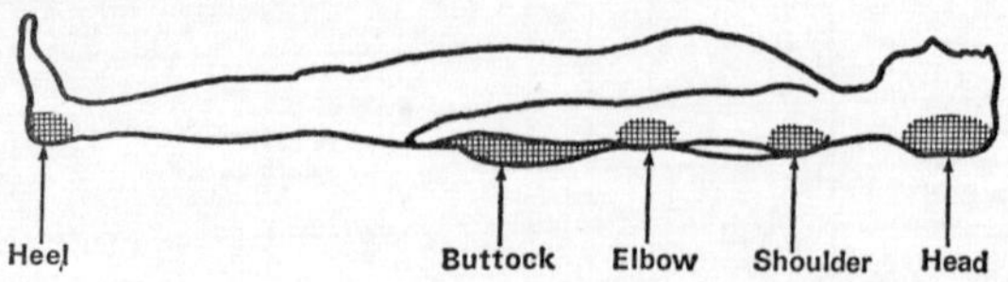

FIG. 17. Common sites of pressure sores.

Deep sores are caused by pressure from the weight of the body in contact with the immovable surface of mattress or chair, causing the tissues to become ischaemic due to an insufficient blood supply. Sustained pressure for long periods is more important than greater pressure for short periods. The deep sore is always found over bony prominences, and the damage occurs initially deep in the muscle and fascia, and spreads to involve breakdown of the skin; when this occurs it may also involve the underlying bone. Initially the skin may only be red and hardened.

It has been shown that the skin is more resistant to the effects of pressure than either the subcutaneous fat or muscle. Moreover, force is often distributed over a wide area of skin surface but the pressure is greatest in the muscle or subcutaneous tissue where the force is concentrated within a small area over a bony prominence. Thus the malignant or deep bedsore starts in the deep tissues.

Superficial sores may occur anywhere on the skin, more commonly in the sacral area, over the spinous processes of the vertebrae, buttocks, elbows, knees and heels. The skin can become damaged by the patient being dragged rather than lifted up the bed or by constant incontinence and of course constant pressure.

It must be remembered that pressure rises with an increase in the inclination of the patient's posture, so that the patient sitting upright is more likely to develop a sacral sore than the recumbent patient. A shearing force, caused by ineffective lifting or by the nurse dragging the patient off the bedpan, damages the blood vessels. Loosely attached superficial fascia slides over well-adhered deep fascia, rupturing the blood vessels. The subcutaneous skin is damaged, causing a haematoma or blister and, if immediate treatment is not efficient, a shallow, painful ulcer may develop. The excoriating effects of the decomposing substances present in urine and infective organisms in faeces are additional hazards. Urea-splitting organisms produce ammonia which causes an alkaline burn, especially if the skin is sodden with moisture.

The majority of sores develop within the first 2 weeks of the patient's stay in hospital, and thus the early days after admission seem to be the time when patients are particularly at risk;

hence the necessity for intensive observation and prophylaxis by the nursing staff.

Prevention

The nurse must always aim to prevent these sores, so prevention will be considered first before treatment of established sores. As the main cause of tissue damage is sustained pressure, the main object of prevention is to relieve pressure.

The two main aetiological factors of poor general condition and immobility are often interrelated. Heart and respiratory disease are liable to increase risk due to poor circulation. Neurological diseases interfere with the nerve supply to the skin and muscle. Incidence is also high in cerebral arteriosclerosis and malignant disease whereas it is low in musculoskeletal disease.

The patient is greatly at risk if he suffers from drowsiness due to over-sedation, poor nutrition, anaemia or urinary, faecal or double incontinence. If some of these conditions are present, help and advice must be sought from the physician. Rest in bed resulting in immobility is usually the commonest complication in the development of a pressure sore, and therefore whenever possible the patient must be encouraged to be ambulant. Early rehabilitation should be aimed at and this may also help to control some incontinence. The underlying causes of the patient's immobility must be investigated and where possible treated by the medical staff, so that the length of stay in bed is reduced to a minimum, and immobility corrected as soon as possible.

Over-sedation should be noted and reported by the nurse, and sedation reduced whenever possible. Poor nutrition may be improved by giving a well-balanced diet specifically qualified with adequate protein and vitamins. It may be complemented with high protein drinks of Casilan and Carnation

Breakfast Food. High potency vitamin supplements are frequently indicated. Anaemia should be corrected and in some cases blood transfusion may be necessary, although if the cause of the anaemia is nutritional or due to malabsorption, the patient will respond to intramuscular iron. It may also be necessary to give oral folic acid and intramuscular cyanocobalamin.

Urinary incontinence may sometimes be improved with drugs and training, and faecal incontinence may nearly always be prevented (see Chapter 4).

Turning the patient Primarily, those patients who are in bed should be turned 2-hourly. Those who have no sores but are at risk should be turned systematically from right lateral to left lateral and, provided they are fully conscious, to the recumbent position. The semi-prone position is not generally tolerated nor comfortable for the elderly patient. In some cases where the skin is extremely fragile, the patient may need turning as often as hourly, but for the fitter patient who is able to move unaided, 4-hourly turning may be adequate. The skin should be washed if the patient is incontinent or sweating, and applications of creams and powders vary according to the individual ward sister's preference.

Local applications There are a large range of preparations for local application to the pressure sore, and this is itself indicative of the lack of knowledge regarding the best preparation. The real danger, irrespective of their individual merits, is reliance on these preparations to the exclusion of knowledge of the patient's condition and the relief of or reduction of pressure.

Reduction of pressure Using an apparatus to record bodily movements during sleep, it has been shown that reduced mobility is directly related to the incidence of pressure sores.

Gentle massage of the pressure points will encourage the circulation in these areas. The natural oil is lost from superficial layers of skin through frequent washing with soap and water, on account of the alkaline content of the soap, and the application of zinc and castor oil cream can help to replace the oil in the incontinent patient. Silicone creams may also be useful as barrier creams to protect the skin. The nurse must be taught to check that the drawsheet contains no rucks, creases or crumbs which can irritate the skin. Occasionally the plastic draw mackintosh causes excessive sweating and may have to be removed.

Those patients at risk must be carefully examined daily and any signs of redness or blisters noted and dealt with accordingly. All patients must be observed for evidence of deterioration in their general condition, and the following points must be observed by the nurse:

Loss of appetite, resulting in inadequate protein intake, reduction in fluid intake leading to dehydration
Signs of confusion
Apathy or drowsiness
Patient becoming unconscious
Development of incontinence

The onset of acute illness will lead to general deterioration and may cause the patient to become temporarily confined to bed.

Although nothing can replace the physical turning of the patient, various devices are available to help the patient, especially at home, and where shortage of nursing staff prevent the highest standard of nursing care being practised.

The large cell *ripple bed* (Fig. 18) manufactured by Talley consists of plastic tubes 10 cm (6 in) in diameter which are alternately filled with air pumped electrically in 10-minute cycles. The tubes may be removed in the appropriate place if the patient has a pressure sore. The small cell ripple bed has proved useful only for very light patients and is now little used.

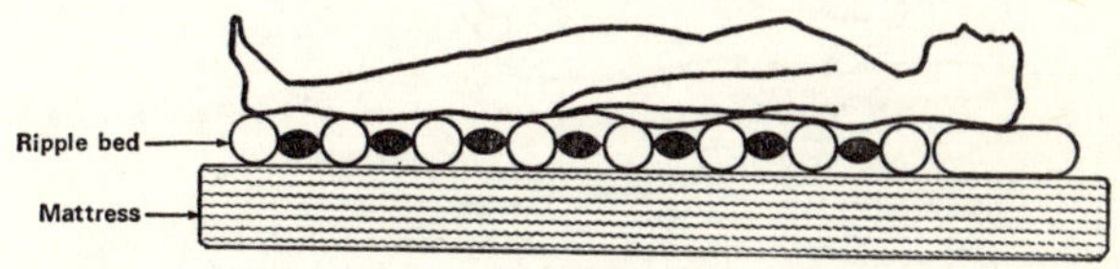

FIG. 18. A large-cell ripple bed.

The Si-rex *air bed* is useful to a degree. It has 2 longitudinal air cells 25 cm (10 in) wide and 3·5 cm (1·5 in) apart, and as the patient moves, so the air moves within the cells and its main use is to facilitate the single-handed turning of an immobile patient. It is obviously less expensive than the Ripple mattress, but it is only 82 cm (33 in) long, thus providing no protection for the heels.

A *water bed* is efficient but very difficult to handle and fill. The experimental water bed manufactured by Beaufort (Air-Sea) Equipment Ltd has proved successful in the treatment of resistant pressure sores. It consists of a water-filled bag of thin nylon restrained by a PVC covered fabric. The patient floats supine on the bed, separated from the water by the thin nylon sheeting which is loosely applied allowing free movement by the patient. The water is maintained at blood heat by an electric heater pumped to and from the bed by an electric pump. Flotation therapy with the patient lying supine ensures that the weight of the body is evenly distributed, with the whole undersurface of the body in contact with the water. The capillary blood flow is not obstructed. The *water pillow*, *air ring* and *Sorbo ring* are all good for protecting the sacral area.

Merino sheepskins (Fig. 19) are useful although not in the case of the incontinent patient, as they would need too

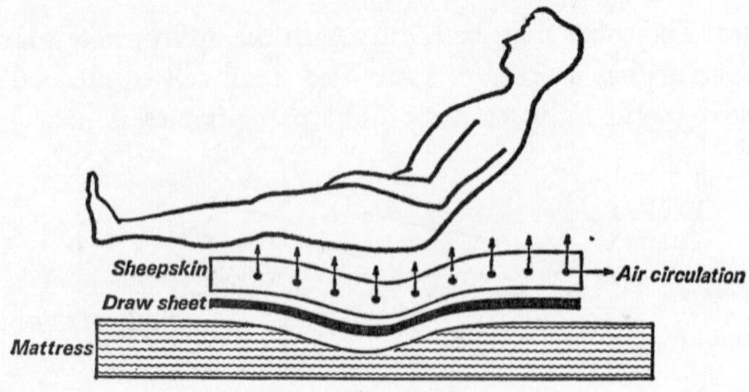

FIG. 19. The sheepskin.

frequent washing. However, experiments in South Africa and New Zealand with sheepskins have proved successful. The natural spring of the wool helps to relieve pressure on the areas of the body in contact with it, the fibres distributing the weight of the patient over a large area and providing an air circulation there, and this also helps to keep the skin dry. Since sheepskin can absorb water up to one-third of its dry weight without feeling wet even patients who perspire freely can benefit from its use. It also prevents friction in the sacral area or wherever else it is used.

The *Alexa-Flote cushion* using flotation techniques is proving useful for protection of the sacrum.

Foam is widely used nowadays, and the Lennard Pad (Fig. 20) or 'cheese' as it is commonly called, has been developed by Professor Brocklehurst for the relief of pressure on the heels. It can be secured in the bed by a draw-sheet, and constant surveillance must be maintained to ensure that, when the patient moves, the wedge is also moved. Foam pads are also useful for relieving pressure between the knees and occasionally for protecting heels and elbows, although the nurse must remove them frequently to check that the skin remains in good condition.

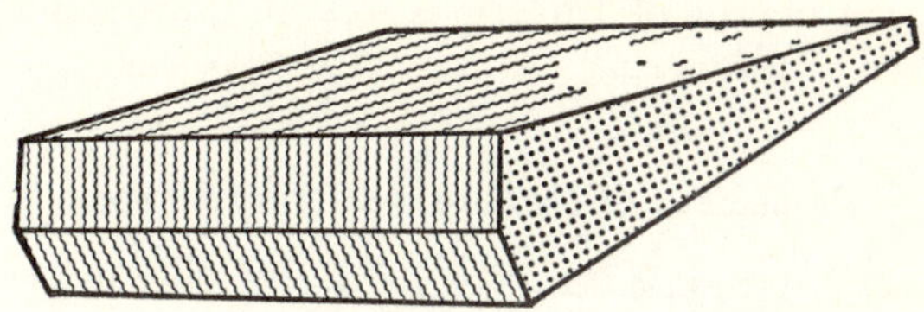

FIG. 20. The Lennard pad.

Heels pose a difficult problem and deep ulcers of the heels are often seen in an otherwise healthy patient. One elderly lady who was severely disabled with arthritis would lie in bed with her heels firmly wedged together. She did this one night, and the foam pad used to separate them was unfortunately omitted. Next morning blisters and a distinct demarcation area appeared. Slowly the two areas broke down but healed again even more slowly. The lady was unable to wear shoes for some time and her walking was somewhat impeded, which was unfortunate, as she needed frequent movement to keep her mobile. The incident illustrates all too well how a slight error of a few hours could cause damage taking days, weeks or even months to correct. The simplest method of protecting heels is to encourage the patient to wear bedsocks. However, if this is done, the patient should be carefully supervised when getting out of bed, as the bedsocks in contact with the floor may cause the patient to slip and fall resulting in possible damage. Should the heels require more protection than this, sheepskin boots may be worn. The cantilever type bed cradle prevents direct pressure on the feet from blankets and also prevents footdrop. A padded footboard reduces the risk of sheering stress. Heel rings and pads are really of limited use and often cause more problems than they solve. If some form of protection is worn, daily inspection of the area must be carried out. Tubipad provides a useful protection for the heels, this is a roll of Tubigrip lined with foam, and may be disposed of after use.

Treatment of Established Pressure Sores

The aim of the nurse here is to promote healing and prevent infection. The patient generally needs to be nursed in bed, therefore rapid healing is desirable so that mobilization is not long delayed. When his general condition improves it may be possible to allow the patient to sit out for short periods, providing no pressure is exerted on the affected area. When a sacral sore is involved, it is sometimes possible to seat the patient in a geriatric chair with the front built up with pillows so that the sacral area is suspended without pressure. It should be remembered that nurses, through a false impression of security, may neglect those severely incapacitated patients confined most of the day to a geriatric chair. They should have the pressure removed from the sacral area for a few minutes every half hour.

The sore usually needs to be dressed 2 or 3 times a day using an aseptic technique. If the sore is only superficial, it may respond well to a daily saline bath, certainly much appreciated by the patient. First all slough must be removed, and this may be done by using eusol or Aserbine lotion or cream; the latter is strong and great care should be exercised to avoid it spreading to the surrounding skin. The surrounding area should be gently massaged to improve the circulation. Ultra-violet light may be used as this aids the de-sloughing of necrotic tissue and stimulates the growth of granulation tissue.

Factors preventing the healing process of a pressure sore include infection, defective oxygenation, oedema, defective nerve supply and continued trauma.

Once the area is clean and healthy, granulation must be encouraged. If possible the area should be exposed to the air, but this may not be practical. Occasionally surgery may be necessary but not often for the geriatric patient. A sinus may develop and lead to infection of underlying bones, and this may have to be opened and drained.

Case History One lady aged only 73 years was admitted with multiple sores. She had taken to her bed a year previously with influenza and had failed to make a complete recovery. Having been looked after by an elderly brother, she had had a completely inadequate diet, and become generally debilitated, doubly incontinent and had developed contractures of both knees. She was a delightful lady who, although she had had a secretarial job throughout her working life, had compensated by such physical activity as playing tennis from the age of 14 to 45. During the treatment of her sores, as described below, she remained totally unaware of her condition and was convinced that she could walk despite severe contractures of both knees; she accepted the sores on her buttocks as being the result of her sedentary work!

Daily saline baths were begun, and fairly rapidly all the superficial sores healed, leaving two deep sinuses on the buttocks, tracking down to the greater trochanter which had become infected. These sinuses had to be opened and drained twice, and were then packed daily with Red lotion dressing, a solution of zinc sulphate which helps in the promotion of healing. The process was very slow.

The general health of a patient must be considered, as sores obviously do not usually occur in those who are healthy and well nourished. Much protein is lost through the established sore and protein is the only foodstuff containing nitrogen which is vital for producing new tissues and replacing waste. A negative nitrogen balance can be avoided by high protein feeding and the use of anabolic agents like Decadurabolin.

Therefore a high protein diet should be given, rich in vitamins, especially vitamin C, which is sometimes given direct to the patient in the form of ascorbic acid.

If the patient is unable to eat normally, a liquid diet should be given reinforced with Casilan and high protein drinks. It may be necessary to pass a nasogastric tube and temporarily feed the patient in this way. Fluids should be encouraged, at least 2 litres per day should be the aim of the nurse.

Antibiotics need rarely be used except when plastic surgery is indicated, or in the case of a diabetic patient, where active and urgent measures need to be taken to prevent extension of the sore. Local antibiotics do not usually prove effective. Some centres have found the application of various forms of syrups and sugars efficient in promoting healing. Obviously prevention of incontinence is essential. Catheterization is indicated if the patient is incontinent of urine, as occasional incontinence especially at night can have a very harmful effect on the cleaning and healing processes. Faecal incontinence must also be controlled.

The complications of pressure sores are many and serious, reinforcing the thesis that prevention is better than cure. Cellulitis, venous thrombosis and emboli may all occur with resulting swelling, inflammation and pain. Bacteraemia may develop which may eventually lead to pyelonephritis, arthritis, meningitis and endocarditis all of which may have very serious complications. Loss of protein and electrolyte imbalance may also occur, and death of the patient may be the eventual outcome of a severe or extensive pressure sore.

7 Nutrition

Studies carried out among the elderly have shown that this section of the population represents the largest single group vulnerable to malnutrition. Elderly house-bound people have been found to have nutrient intakes which are substantially lower than those of active people of comparable age.

Malnutrition can be defined as 'the condition in which nutrition is defective in quantity or quality'. The condition includes both under-nutrition and obesity. As Cheyne said in 1725, 'most of all chronic diseases, the infirmities of old age and the short period of the lives of English men are owing to repletion'. Obesity usually results from lifelong faulty eating habits, and in this respect differs from under-nutrition which often arises from environmental and physical factors operating for the first time in later life.

Changes in physical activity, body composition and efficiency of muscular movements probably cause little deterioration in the total gross metabolism of the body with ageing, but primary causes of malnutrition in the elderly include ignorance, social isolation, physical disability, mental disturbance and poverty. Secondary causes include impaired appetite, inability to masticate properly and malabsorption. These will be discussed further later in the chapter.

The energy value of foods is measured in heat units—calories—which provide an assessment of the amounts of food required by different people in accordance with their age, build and occupation. The chief broad groups of foods will provide the following values in calories:

1 g carbohydrate (as glucose)	3·75 calories
1 g fat	9·3 calories
1 g protein	4·1 calories

The normal calorie requirements of an elderly man upon retirement are approximately 2300 per day and should stay at this level as long as he remains active; the basal requirement may be only 1500 calories. For women the requirement is 2000–1500 calories and the basal requirement 1250.

First the nurse must be familiar with the basic constituents of food and their actions. Present knowledge of the influence of ageing on the quantity of food eaten and energy expenditure is deficient, and further investigations are needed in this field.

Carbohydrates

These are small sugar molecules composed of carbon, hydrogen and oxygen. They are transported in the blood stream and are converted into carbon dioxide and water, releasing some energy as heat, the remainder being stored in the form of glycogen in the liver and cells, being used as necessary to maintain a chemical balance and for physical activity. A certain concentration of glucose is maintained in the blood by the liver and varies between 80 and 150 mg/100 ml.

Sources: fruit, sugar, potatoes, flour, bread, rice.

Excess intake causes obesity and digestive disorders. Lack of carbohydrate can lead to ketosis, when fat is used for the production of energy to a greater extent than normal. The majority of elderly people have a high intake of carbohydrates as they are found in the less expensive forms of food and need little preparation.

Cellulose consists of large molecules of carbohydrate which cannot be split and pass unaltered through the alimentary tract. Cellulose is contained in fruit and vegetables and, since they stimulate peristalsis of the bowel, these help to establish regular bowel habits.

Fat

Although fat has the same constituents as glucose, it can release more energy per unit weight. Any excess fat is stored in the fat deposits in the body, mainly subcutaneously and around the abdominal organs. Fat is a component of cell membranes and is particularly important with regard to the cells of the nervous system.

Sources: butter, meat, milk, some fish, lard, vegetable oils and nut oils when converted into margarine.

There is some relation between fats and arterial disease in which fatty materials are deposited in the arterial walls, but no absolute recommendation about diets in this respect seems justifiable for this age group. However, it is important in early years to reduce the incidence of cerebrovascular disease, myocardial infarction, peripheral vascular disease and diabetes mellitus, by exercising care with the quantity of fats consumed.

Protein

Protein is a principal constituent of every living cell. Protein is composed of carbon, hydrogen, oxygen and nitrogen, and is the only food source of nitrogen for the body. It consists of amino acids of which there are known to be 23.

Some protein is lost to the body during metabolism and amino acids from the diet are necessary for replacement. Amino acids are required by the tissues for the production of enzymes, hormones, haemoglobin and antibodies. Protein is also a source of energy.

Sources: animal protein such as meat, fish, cheese, eggs and milk; vegetable protein such as green peas, lentils, peanuts, baked beans.

Studies have shown that women with high protein intake enjoy better health than those with low intake. The daily intake should not fall with age and should be 1 g/kg of body weight per day. There is an increased need in debilitating illness and conditions with excessive loss, for example severe pressure sores; this may be assisted by the use of anabolic steroids.

Protein, particularly meat, is an expensive form of food and therefore not always eaten in sufficient quantities. Cheese is not popular with the elderly, but milk is widely consumed. Bread contains a certain amount of protein, and many elderly people obtain as much as 20% of their protein from this source.

Vitamins

Fat-soluble Vitamins

Vitamin A This is essential for normal vision and maintains the epithelial tissue of the body. Deficiency, rarely seen in the elderly, results in night-blindness and infections of the mucous membranes.

Sources: meat, fish, fish oils, butter, cheese.

Vitamin K This is essential for the formation of prothrombin in the liver which is required for the clotting of blood. There is no evidence of deficiency in the elderly except in obstructive jaundice when lack of bile salts will impair absorption.

Source: green vegetables.

Vitamin D This increases the absorption of calcium and phosphorus from the digestive tract and promotes the deposition on the bone. Deficiency in children causes rickets and in the elderly produces evidence of osteomalacia which may be symptomless unless a fracture occurs. There may be evidence of general muscular weakness, a waddling gait, difficulty with stairs, low backache, stiffness and bone tenderness. The results of deficiency of vitamin D include malabsorption, post-gastrectomy syndrome, liver and kidney disease. Much of the body's requirement is met by synthesis in the skin by ultra-violet light in the form of sunlight often missed by the elderly.

Sources: eggs, fish, margarine, sunlight.

Water-soluble Vitamins

Vitamin B This is a complex of different vitamins: thiamine, riboflavine, niacine, pyridoxine, pantotheric acid, biotin, folic acid and cyanocobalamin.

Vitamin B1 Thiamine constitutes part of an enzyme system concerned in the metabolism of carbohydrate. Deficiency is believed to be the principal cause of beri-beri which occurs among people whose staple food is polished rice, since thiamine is found in the discarded husks of the rice. Such deficiency results in polyneuritis which involves the legs and feet, and causes pain and weakness, and inability to coordinate. In Great Britain, deficiency of vitamin B1 is thought to cause acute confusional states and neuritis amongst elderly people.

Source: wholemeal flour and bread, liver.

Riboflavin This is essential for tissue oxidation. Deficiency results in glossitis and dermatitis round the mouth, nose, vulva and scrotum. Deficiency is rare in this country.

Source: Milk, liver, kidneys, heart and egg yolk.

Niacin or nicotinic acid This has similar action to riboflavine. Deficiency, along with other vitamins of the B complex, causes pellagra. Reddish-brown areas appear on the skin, especially the neck, face and hands. Dermatitis, diarrhoea and dementia may also occur.

Source: yeast, wholemeal bread, liver, meat.

Pyridoxine This has an important action in amino acid metabolism. Deficiency leads to mental confusion, depression and dermatitis.

Source: yeast, liver, wheat, corn.

Vitamin B12 or cyanocobalamin This is the extrinsic factor necessary for normal red cell maturation, but it cannot be absorbed without the intrinsic factor present in gastric secretions. Deficiency is quite often found in the elderly who lack the intrinsic factor necessary for absorption due to impairment of gastric secretions and the patient develops Addisonian or pernicious anaemia, named after Addison of Guy's Hospital who described the condition in 1855. The onset is gradual and therefore symptoms may not present until the haemoglobin is below 6 g/100 ml. The patient may complain of breathlessness, weakness and swollen ankles; the skin has a yellow or lemon tint. Treatment is to give intramuscular injections of cyanocobalamin daily initially, then weekly and eventually monthly for the rest of their lives.

Subacute combined degeneration of the spinal cord is closely associated with Addisonian anaemia. The patient complains of numbness in the feet and fingers, weakness and unsteadiness when walking. The treatment is similar to that of Addisonian anaemia, but the cyanocobalamin is given more frequently initially and in larger doses.

Source: liver, kidney, heart, fish, cheese, eggs.

Folic acid This, like vitamin B12, is necessary for the development of red blood corpuscles and maturation of the nuclei. Deficiency occurs when the elderly have disorders of the gastrointestinal tract giving rise to malabsorption. It may be replaced in oral form.

Source: green leafy vegetables.

Vitamin C This is necessary for the formation of red cells and the absorption of iron. It is also required for the metabolism of amino acids, and the formation of collagen in connective tissue, and is thus necessary for sound healing of wounds.

Vitamin C is the most easily destroyed vitamin, although it is less easily destroyed in dried foods. In homes and hospitals where there is bulk cooking and vegetables tend to be cooked for too long and then kept warm for several hours before delivering them to the patient, there is a real risk of vitamin C deficiency. The most common vegetables are potatoes and cabbage. To retain the maximum amount of vitamin C the vegetables should be cooked unpeeled if possible and in large pieces so that water-soluble nutrients are not lost through the cut surfaces. As little water as possible should be used and they should be cooked for the shortest possible time and served immediately. Ascorbic acid is easily destroyed by heat and exposure to light.

Deficiency causes weakness, irritability, decreased resistance to infection and pains in the limbs and joints. Prolonged deficiency causes scurvy when there are multiple haemorrhages, swollen painful gums, haemorrhages into the joints and degenerative changes of the bones.

Source: citrus fruit such as oranges, lemons, grapefruit; tomatoes; leafy vegetables; soft fruits such as blackcurrants, gooseberries, raspberries, strawberries. Potatoes have a small, but important, amount as they are the staple food of many who cannot afford the more expensive fruit.

Case history Mr X., aged 82, was admitted from home thought to be deficient in vitamin C. His wife had died 2 years previously, and although he had managed well at first, he had gradually sunk into a state of apathy and was existing on tinned rice pudding. He was edentulous but his gums did appear swollen, he was very irritable and obstreperous at times, he had a few petechial haemorrhages and unhealed varicose ulcers on both legs which were heavily infected and neglected. Mr X. commenced large doses of ascorbic acid, 100 g three times daily; he was also given a nutritious but soft diet, rich in protein, and wherever possible fresh fruit. The infections of his legs were treated and slowly the ulcers began to heal. Several months later Mr X. was fit enough to leave hospital and he agreed reluctantly to leave his home, and live in council residential accommodation. He never would agree to see a dentist!

Calcium

This is the mineral which occurs in the greatest amount in the body and is the structural component of bone. It is absorbed from the alimentary tract with the aid of vitamin D. Deficiency results in osteoporosis, a common disorder in elderly persons, especially women. There is a reduction of the bone mass with a change in the constitution. The bones become radiologically less dense and clinically more brittle. The most notable symptom of the disease is pain. There is sometimes kyphosis and loss of height but many patients have also compression fractures of the vertebral bodies. The treatment and progress are slow. Calcium can be given orally and can be enhanced by giving anabolic steroids, e.g. Durabolin. A spinal support may be necessary and helpful.

Source: milk and cheese are the main sources. Milk has a high content, is easily available, relatively inexpensive and a staple food.

Iron

Iron is necessary for the formation of haemoglobin which is a constituent of the red blood cells. Haemoglobin is responsible for the transportation of oxygen and carbon dioxide between the lungs and the tissues. Only a small quantity of iron is absorbed from food and this is facilitated by ascorbic acid and possibly hydrochloric acid, as iron deficiency is usually present when there is an achlorhydria (absence of hydrochloric acid in the stomach). Achlorhydria is common in old age hence this might explain the malabsorption of iron resulting in iron deficiency anaemia. Also the elderly tend to suffer from minor gastrointestinal haemorrhages with chronic loss of blood.

It has been found difficult to maintain the iron content of hospital diets at an acceptable level, so it must be much more difficult for the elderly living alone on restricted incomes.

Source: meat, especially liver, eggs, green leafy vegetables, fish, wholemeal flour and bread.

Fluid Requirements

The elderly person requires approximately 2 litres of liquid every 24 hours, and this should be increased if fever, sweating, polyuria or dehydration are present. If eating normally, the patient will ingest 1 litre of fluid in his food but if not 2 litres must be provided in fluids.

Frequently it is very difficult to persuade elderly patients to drink this amount, especially women who do not wish to be disturbed at night or fear to wet the bed. Many find it a great effort to drink when ill, and some have difficulty in swallowing.

Causes of Malnutrition

The most common cause of malnutrition is inadequate diet, for which there are a variety of causes.

1. The elderly person may live alone, thus having no incentive to cook adequate meals.

2. The elderly person may live alone and have difficulty shopping, cooking, and preparing food because of physical disability, e.g. those with arthritis, parkinsonism and following a cerebrovascular accident.

3. The elderly man, living alone following the death of his wife, finds he cannot manage to feed himself adequately.

4. Depression in the elderly may cause loss of appetite leading to a general deterioration and malnutrition.

5. The elderly person living on a very small income cannot afford the correct foods and is unaware of the financial benefits available within the welfare state. The more desirable foods are not only more expensive, but take more time and trouble to cook as well as being perishable.

All these people may benefit from various facilities available to help them:

1. Luncheon Clubs, usually run by the Women's Royal Voluntary Service once or twice a week, where a balanced meal can be enjoyed in a congenial atmosphere.

2. A day club or day centre usually run by Age Concern in a town, again where good food can be enjoyed in good company, and some people may be able to attend several times a week. This may help to correct the inadequate diet received at home.

3. Meals-on-Wheels, prepared and delivered by the Women's Royal Voluntary Service, are provided 2 or 3 times a week and help to provide a nutritious meal on these occasions, thus supplementing an otherwise inadequate diet.

4. The Home-Help service, organized by the Social Services Department of the Local Authority, aims to provide someone to cook a meal regularly in the elderly person's home where this is necessary. This person will also shop and thus see that there is food in the house in the interim period.

Feeding in Hospital

Meals should be small and well presented, and, where possible, the patient should be provided with what he feels he can eat. Some may not be able to eat solid food because they lack natural teeth or cannot use ill-fitting artificial teeth. Puréed foods are usually available and Heinz baby purées are often appreciated by these people. A liquidizer on the ward is an advantage and widens the scope of meals. Use should be made of Complan and Carnation Breakfast Foods. The latter has several different flavours and is quite palatable; it has quite a high protein content and this may be enhanced by the addition of a beaten egg.

It is important that the patient be placed in the most comfortable position for meals, so that he can enjoy them and wherever possible feed himself. Only when really necessary should the patient be fed as this is a very degrading process. Where feeding is necessary the nurse should be seated, give the patient her full attention and appear not to be in a hurry.

Various aids are available for helping the handicapped patient to eat. If the patient is severely handicapped, he will be assessed by the occupational therapist and the most suitable implements provided. Those who experience the most problems when feeding are the patients who suffer from severe arthritis, hemiplegia following a cerebrovascular accident and Parkinson's disease.

Non-slip mats are useful if the eating surface is slippery; plate bunkers and bowls produced in the Manoy range of Melaware are also very useful. There are also various pieces of cutlery adapted for the disabled.

Help should be enlisted from the dietician for those who require special diets, and she should see that the patient has received adequate instruction and advice before being discharged from hospital.

Intragastric Feeding

The unconscious patient must be fed by an intragastric tube, a suitable diet having been devised. Feeds are generally given 2-hourly during the day and less frequently at night. A fluid intake of 2 litres should be adequate unless there are contra-indications requiring more or less fluid. The calorific value is worked out according to the patient's needs.

Passing a Nasogastric Tube

The tube is usually passed and left in situ, being changed 2 or 3 times a week. The patient will be placed in the recumbent position with the head raised and tilted forward. If the patient is conscious a clear explanation will be given by the nurse before starting the procedure. The tube is passed through the nostril to the stomach, and if the patient is cooperative he can be asked to swallow at the appropriate time. If the tube should enter either bronchus, the patient will immediately cough or become cyanosed and the tube must be withdrawn at once. When the tube is in place the nurse must check with a registered nurse that it is in fact in the correct position. This can be done by aspirating part of the stomach content and testing it for acidity, or placing a funnel on the end of the tube and inverting it in some water. If the tube is in the bronchus bubbles will be seen and the water will rise and fall in the funnel on inspiration and expiration. The tube is then secured in position with some adhesive tape and a spigot placed in the end.

Before giving a feed, the patient will be turned on his side so that if he vomits, he will not inhale his vomit. He should always be turned before not after the feed, as turning on a full stomach may cause the patient to vomit. The tube should be checked before every feed, as it is very easy for it to enter the trachea without causing any distress to the patient. The feed should be given at a temperature of 37°C (98·5°F) and slowly so as not to overload the stomach.

On admission to hospital, the elderly patient is often dehydrated and requires rehydration before treatment for the specific disease can begin. It is often far more beneficial to the patient to give intravenous fluids for 24–48 hours than to struggle with oral fluids for the reluctant drinker. The intravenous fluids will be prescribed by the doctor and will also correct the electrolyte imbalance which may have occurred. Intravenous feeding may be necessary for some time for those patients who cannot tolerate food by mouth or nasogastric tube. This is an expensive form of feeding which is also very irritable to the vein and is only used when no other form of feeding is possible.

Carbohydrate is given as fructose or glucose and the most common is 30% sorbitol, supplying 1200 calories per litre. Fat emulsion is derived from cotton seed oil and soya bean oil. One litre of 10% fat emulsion, with the addition of 5% sorbitol to render it isotonic, will provide 1780 calories.

Protein is provided in the form of amino acids. These are usually combined in one preparation which combines amino acids and fructose and provides 875 calories per litre.

In many cases it may be necessary to keep an accurate fluid balance chart. Fluid intake and output should be measured and charted. The chart should be kept in an obvious place and all members of the staff should be aware of it.

Obesity

Obesity is a more common disease than undernutrition, especially among women, and is more usually seen in the less wealthy or less well informed people who become obese because their diet consists of too much carbohydrate and too little protein, fruit and green vegetables. Carbohydrate tends to be found in the less expensive types of food which need little preparation. There are many other causes such as lack of mobility due to degenerative diseases common in old age, familial tendencies, endocrine factors, the habit of taking snacks between meals, and the greatest factor is the life-long habit of overeating, possibly as a consequence of boredom and a refuge from unhappiness. Some people in middle age tend to regard overweight at this period of their lives as a sign of good health.

Complications

Many people who develop diabetes in middle age or beyond are overweight and have a tendency to be obese. There is increased likelihood of fatty degeneration of the heart, hypertension and angina occurring. Heart failure may result with dependent oedema and leg ulceration. Chronic bronchitis and emphysema is more common in the obese and surgery, especially abdominal operations, is often more difficult and leads to complications. The most common and most disabling complication of obesity is degenerative arthritis of the weight-bearing joints.

Mobility is obviously reduced and the patient is at a grave disadvantage when requiring rehabilitation after a fracture or a cerebrovascular accident. If confined to bed, the patient is far more likely to develop a pressure sore, deep vein thrombosis or pulmonary embolism. These patients cause extra stress on their families and nurses when they become ill and require nursing.

It is most important that people should be educated early concerning the dangers of obesity in later life.

Weight-reducing Programme

This allows an intake of approximately 1000 calories

Daily allowance	½ pt (500 ml) milk ½ oz (14 g) butter *or* margarine 3 oz (85 g) bread
Breakfast	Fresh grapefruit *or* small orange *or* 4 oz (120 ml) unsweetened fruit juice (small glass) 1 egg, boiled or poached *or* 1 oz (28 g) grilled bacon (1 rasher) Tomato *or* mushrooms, as liked 1 oz (28 g) bread Scraping of butter (*or* margarine) from allowance Tea *or* coffee, with milk from allowance
Mid-morning	Tea *or* coffee, with milk from allowance *or* Bovril *or* Oxo *or* Marmite
Dinner at midday or evening	3 oz (84 g) lean meat with unthickened gravy *or* 5 oz (140 g) fish Green vegetables, as liked Root vegetables (e.g. carrot, beetroot) 1 tablespoon 1 portion fresh or stewed fruit
Mid-afternoon	1 oz (28 g) bread Scraping of butter (*or* margarine) from allowance Salad vegetable *or* Marmite Tea with milk from allowance
Supper or lunch	3 oz (84 g) lean meat with unthickened gravy *or* 5 oz (140 g) fish *or* 1½ oz (42 g) cheese *or* 2 eggs Green vegetables *or* salad, as liked 1 oz (28 g) bread Scraping of butter (*or* margarine) from allowance 1 portion fresh or stewed fruit
Bedtime	Tea *or* coffee, with milk from allowance *or* Bovril *or* Oxo *or* Marmite

Anorexiogenic agents are of little value in these elderly obese patients. They only have their use in those who have recently become overweight or for those who have had repeated failures or attempts to lose weight.

It is essential to have the patient's whole cooperation and that of the family. It is pointless placing the patient on a diet if the family bring in biscuits, cakes and sweets every time they visit. If everyone has a full explanation of the complications of obesity, there is more hope of a good result.

The patient may be given a 1000 calorie diet with the help of the dietician and supplements of iron, calcium and vitamins are essential. The patient should be weighed regularly under similar conditions to make sure that weight is being lost and to give encouragement.

Thus it can be seen that, although both over- and under-nourishment are encountered in the geriatric unit, over-nourishment has far longer lasting and more serious side-effects.

8 Rehabilitation

Rehabilitation is very much an exercise in team work, and the successful outcome of the patient's treatment depends upon the ability of the members of the team to work well together. The leader of the team must obviously be the physician in charge, and the work is shared amongst the nursing staff, occupational therapists, physiotherapists, speech therapists and social workers. In some units rehabilitation aides may also be used. These are people trained specifically in rehabilitation who work within the departments and the wards. Important members of the team also are the porters and ambulance drivers who transport the patients and play a big part in making their visit enjoyable, and also the chiropodist, because unless the patient's feet are well cared for, he is unable even to attempt to walk. In order to work more closely with these people the nurse must understand the principles of the therapists' work.

The Occupational Therapist

The occupational therapist assesses the functional disability of the patient in relation to the activities of daily living, watching the patient dressing, getting in and out of bed, off the lavatory, in and out of the bath, cooking and washing up. She will advise and give assistance where necessary, and will teach the patient how best to cope with his or her disability. She will also teach the relatives how they can best manage the patient's problems when the time comes for him to go home, and they may come and spend a day in the occupational therapy department. None of this can be done unless the occupational therapist has knowledge of the patient's home conditions. She may visit the home to assess the situation and to determine whether there is need for any alterations or improvements. She will note whether the patient has a chair, bed and lavatory at the right height and, where there are stairs, whether it will be possible for the patient to get up and down them.

The occupational therapist also provides and supervises exercises for specific disabilities. For instance, various forms of basket-making provide exercises for the joints of the hands and fingers. Weaving and loom work teach coordination of hands and eyes and provide some arm work, and working on large looms involves arms and legs also.

The therapist will want to know what goal the patient is aiming for, so this must be clearly defined by the whole team, and if necessary a time limit must be set so that everyone is aware of the objective. Group activities will also be included in her work, and these enable the patient to communicate with others and give a sense of purpose and belonging.

The Physiotherapist

Regular physiotherapy is not only valuable but indeed essential treatment in the majority of diseases encountered on the geriatric ward, e.g. patients suffering from cerebrovascular accident with resulting hemiplegia, Parkinsonism, varicose ulcers, arthritis, fracture and amputation.

The physiotherapist must firstly assess the patient's condition and teach him how to become mobile again, providing him with a suitable aid as necessary. Once he has learned to walk again, he can quickly regain much more independence. Secondly, the physiotherapist is concerned with maintenance of function in those patients with a long-standing disability such as osteoarthrosis, who developed another condition such as diabetes or heart failure, which may require a period of investigation and even immobilization in hospital. This may result in weakness or contractures and loss of former mobility. Thirdly the physiotherapist may also give specific exercises for various disabilities and disuse of muscles and joints. She may be required to give infra-red heat and ultra-violet light for specific lesions.

Her work is closely aligned to that of the occupational therapist, but the nursing staff must also work with her as they must carry on the patient's treatment in the absence of the physiotherapist. All members of the nursing staff must be aware of the patient's capabilities, and what aids and how many people are required to help the patient walk or transfer from bed to chair. There should be some form of indication in writing of this (Kardex, for example) somewhere in the ward to which all can refer, thus avoiding confusion.

The Speech Therapist

The speech therapist concentrates on the patient with speech defects, generally following cerebrovascular accident or where there is a cerebral lesion. She will work with the patients individually and in groups to help them overcome their disabilities and learn to communicate again with those around them.

When the speech therapist is working on the wards the nurse must allow her a quiet corner so that the patient is not distracted by noise and activity around her, and can concentrate fully on the training.

The Social Worker

The social worker has an important function in the team while the patient is being rehabilitated. She must cooperate with all the staff and attend to the patient's financial and home commitments, and allay any fears concerning these that may arise. She liaises between staff and relatives to see that suitable clothes and shoes are available for the patient. She will also assist in the patient's future. She will help organize the home if necessary to see that all is ready for the patient's return and liaise with the social services department of the local authority if any alterations need to be made. If the patient is unable to return home and suitable accommodation must be found, application may have to be made to the local authority for residential accommodation. In this case the patient must be fitted into a suitable home where the staff can meet the

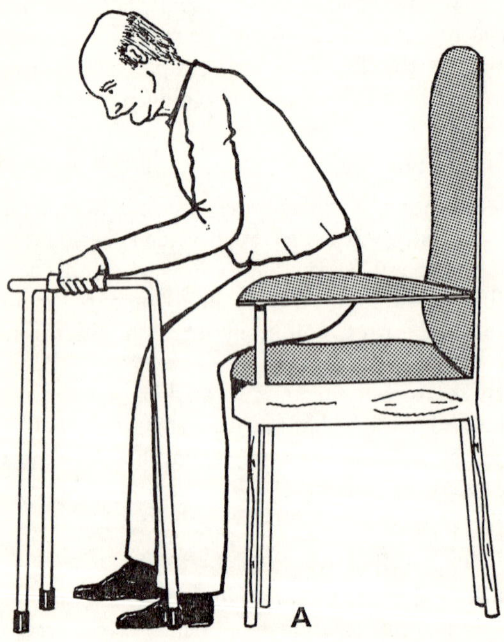

FIG. 21. The incorrect (A) and correct (B, facing) way for an elderly patient to rise from a chair.

patient's needs, and the patient will find congenial company, and both he and his relatives are happy in the arrangement.

General Principles of Rehabilitation

The general principles of rehabilitation may be summarized as maintaining and improving the mobility of the patient's joints, preserving and improving the muscle power, and actively restoring and developing muscle function. While all this is in progress, especially for the elderly patient, it is necessary to maintain and improve their morale, which is

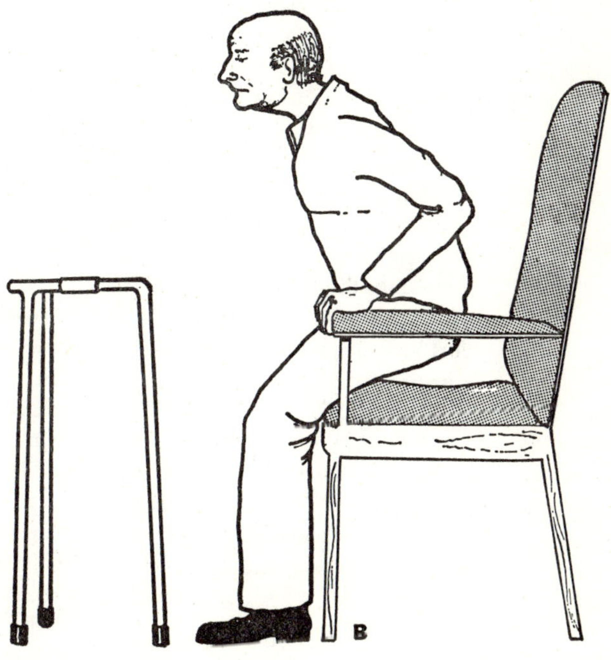

obviously low on admission to hospital, for the other work to be effective.

The requirements of a successful rehabilitation unit are plenty of space and a well trained staff, and success depends upon maximal patient cooperation with the patient becoming the central member of the team.

It is the nurse's responsibility to see that the ground which the patient has gained in a short period of treatment with one of the rehabilitation specialists, the physiotherapist or occupational therapist, is extended during the rest of the patient's day and at the weekend. Most nurses now receive some training from the physiotherapist in the basic techniques of transferring a patient from bed to chair, from chair to commode. They learn the correct way to help a patient up from a chair on to a walking aid, and the importance of ensuring that he has got his balance before he moves off (Fig. 21). The nurse can learn from the physiotherapist the way to prevent a frozen shoulder in a hemiplegic patient, simply by elevating the patient's weak arm whenever she attends to him for any reason.

Similarly with dressing, the detailed assessment of a patient with a dressing disability takes a very long time and is primarily work for the occupational therapist. But as the patient improves the work can be taken over by the nurse. She can assist him by seeing that his clothes are in proper order. She must not retard his progress by taking over the whole job herself in order to save time unless he is completely helpless.

First the patient must be assessed as to his physical disabilities and also to his possible capabilities. There should be frequent discussion between the physician, therapists, social worker and nursing staff, as to the limits to which rehabilitation should be pursued. After assessment and a period of intensive rehabilitation it may be necessary for an aid to be supplied. This is usually prescribed by the consultant if he decides that the patient is unable to manage without such help. When this is so, acceptance of the aid depends upon an early decision to use it, its efficiency and the understanding, motivation and cooperation of the patient in learning to use it.

Appliances

An appliance is a device made to fit the patient in order to correct a deformity or increase a function, e.g. corsets, calipers, surgical footwear and splints.

Corsets are often supplied in cases of osteoporosis and osteoarthrosis of the spine, giving good support, and helping the patient when walking, possibly relieving pain when sitting.

Calipers are sometimes required by patients following a cerebrovascular accident and in cases of footdrop and peroneal weakness which may occur after surgery or prolonged bed rest. These are usually only prescribed after a period of intensive rehabilitation, as considerable functional improvement may occur with exercise.

Surgical footwear consisting of boots and shoes is generally supplied to those with ankle weakness due to hemiplegia, severe osteoarthrosis, rheumatoid arthritis and foot deformities.

Splints may be required for the arthritic or hemiplegic patient to ensure good position during periods of bed rest and enforced rest. In the case of the patient with rheumatoid arthritis, it may be necessary to rest the joint concerned for some time until the inflammation subsides. Occasionally when weakness of the wrist occurs, it may be necessary to use a splint for stabilization to help the patient to feed independently.

Personal aids These consist of small items to assist functional ability, e.g. pick up sticks, bath aids, toilet aids, eating aids, household gadgets and adapted clothing. Most of these are only given after considerable assessment and active exercises as they can result in ultimate lessening of function, and if this function can be maintained for a little longer, it is ultimately to the patient's advantage.

Washing and Bathing

Many patients can manage to wash partially without assistance, but the nurse may well need to give help to wash feet, backs and perineal area. For many of the elderly, baths are dangerous and should not be attempted alone at home without help from the home nurse or a relative. So often the patient finds he can get into the bath quite easily, but cannot get out alone. A shower is a suitable form of toilet for the elderly, although not often appreciated by this generation.

Bath aids These consist of various seats that enable the patient to get in and out without too much difficulty, and to lower themselves into the bath slowly. There are also various rails which can be fixed by the local authority to enable safer entry and exit to the bath.

Lavatory aids These are a variety of rails and seat raises which can easily be fixed, as most patients find difficulty in rising from the modern rather low lavatory.

Clothing

Adapted clothing is often very necessary and much is now readily available. Geriatric dresses with slits down the side or back and a fly-away panel are on the market, and are usually made of easily washable material needing no ironing. They are much easier to manage than pulling up a tight skirt or trying to sit elegantly in such a skirt. Similarly, trousers are made in Terylene, which is easy to wash, and have a Velcro fastening.

Shoes may prove a problem as leather may become stiff and hard due to incontinence of urine. However, there are various synthetic lace-up shoes now available which are also washable and wear reasonably well. Various other garments may be adapted by the occupational therapists to various patients' individual needs, as no two people have the same disabilities and precise difficulties.

Equipment

This consists of larger mechanical aids, hoists, special beds, adapted kitchen equipment, special chairs and remote control equipment such as the POSSUM which can control door opening, television, wireless, tape recorder and typewriter amongst its functions. All this is very expensive equipment, and responsibility for its supply rests with the consultant and the social services department of the local authority. The discretionary powers of local authorities are very wide-ranging, from provision of personal aids to architectural reconstruction of the patient's home, building ramps, widening doors and installing hoists. Financial arrangements vary considerably from authority to authority as does the ease with which aids are available.

The practical application of the principles of good rehabilitation can usefully be illustrated by studying a case history.

Case history Mrs B., aged 82 years, was admitted from home having collapsed that morning. She was conscious but drowsy and had evidence of a right hemiparesis, having a little movement in her arm and leg. That evening she was seen by the physiotherapist and some active and passive movements were carried out on the patient's arms and legs. While in bed the affected limbs were kept in a good position, and a bed cradle and padded footboard were also placed in the bed to prevent footdrop.

During the next 2 days Mrs B. appeared to be making good progress and was able to sit in a chair for short periods. She had only minimal weakness in her leg and her balance was good, and the nurses were able to teach her the correct way to transfer from bed to chair. From the beginning she always wore a good pair of lace-up shoes which her daughter had

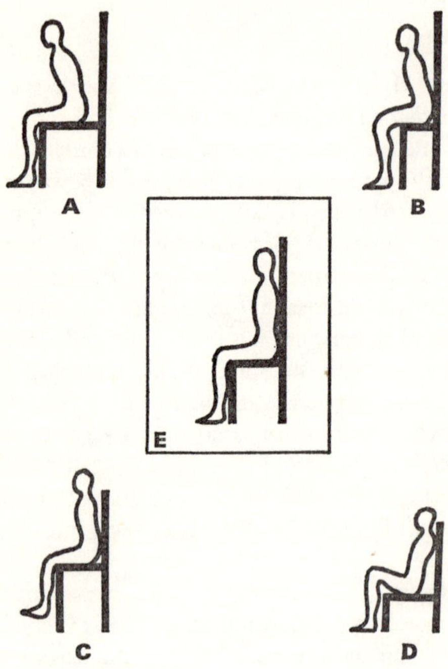

FIG. 22. Suitable and unsuitable chairs. A, Seat too broad. B, Seat too narrow. C, Too high. D, Too low. E, A good fit.

brought in for her. There appeared to be very little movement in her arm and the physiotherapist taught her various exercises which she could do while sitting in a chair. A suitable chair (Fig. 22) was provided with a straight back and arms, so that the patient could get up without too much difficulty. The ward needs to have a variety of geriatric chairs, as different chairs suit different patients; some require a higher chair than others and some appreciate a foot rest, while the more active no longer have need of this. To ensure maximum independence also the bed needs to be of a suitable height, so that the patient is able to get in and out unaided if possible.

When Mrs B. began to walk, she needed the support of two members of staff, usually the physiotherapist and a nurse, but the staff felt that it was essential that she became independent as soon as possible, and this was done by providing her with a quadriped which she soon learnt to use, firstly with an aide and then managing to walk alone.

Walking is dependent on the strength and endurance of the patient. Difficulty in walking may occur in various diseases. The hemiplegic patient may experience difficulties due to interference of balance, muscle weakness and spasticity. Balance may be disturbed as a result of lesions of the cerebellar system or visual impairment. There may be weakness of the muscles of the trunk, abdomen, hip, knee or foot groups, and all these may have an effect on walking.

Some patients do not progress well with walking and may be considered for a wheelchair after all other efforts to get the patient mobile have failed. Sometimes an ordinary small wheelchair may be sufficient for a relative to push the patient longer distances. Self-propelled wheelchairs are available with aid wheels on both or either side depending upon the handicap. The chairs have to be carefully fitted according to the patient's measurements and disability. For those with a severe disability an electric wheelchair may be necessary with convenient hand controls. When a wheelchair is considered, the home must also be examined to ensure that this is practicable there, and to see whether any alterations need to be made to accommodate the chair.

However, Mrs B. managed well with her quadriped; all the

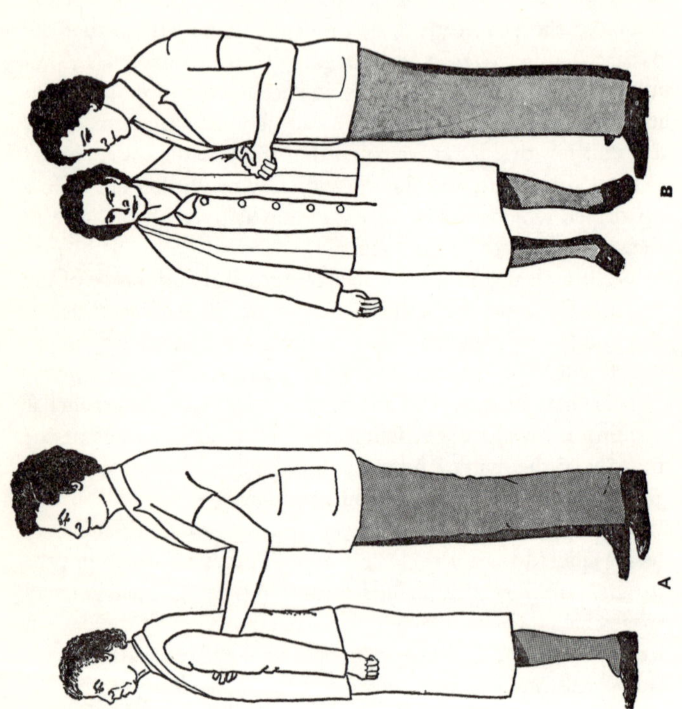

FIG. 23. The incorrect (A) and correct (B) way to walk a patient.

nursing staff knew that she could use this aid and that she was considered safe to walk alone. While Mrs B. was learning to walk, she was also learning to use the lavatory unaided, to feed and dress herself. The nurse, physiotherapist and occupational therapist all worked together and Mrs B. attended the occupational therapy department 2 or 3 mornings per week to pursue her activities. Mrs B. was encouraged to be dressed in her own clothes early on during her stay, as this has a remarkable effect on the patient's morale. The daughter was advised to bring in dresses which had easy access, as Mrs B. still had little movement in her right arm, making dressing a difficult procedure.

Mrs B. did have some problems when eating and drinking as she had to manage this left-handed. She was never encouraged to be fed, as this can be very degrading and frustrating for the patient. She found it much easier to manage when sitting in a chair, and was therefore always up for supper and breakfast. Sometimes the diet can be adapted to the benefit of the patient and help may be obtained from the dietician and catering officer, e.g. salads are difficult to manage unless shredded, soups are easier to manage if they are thicker and can be drunk from a cup rather than from a bowl. Mrs B. was provided with a Nelson knife which incorporated a cutting device and a fork. The staff always ensured that her plate was placed on a non-slip mat, so she did not have to worry about it sliding about the table, and she always had a plate bunker or Manoy bowl, so that she did not have to chase the food round the plate thus allowing it to become unnecessarily cold.

Speech

The speech therapist may be treating patients with speech difficulties only usually occurring following a cerebrovascular accident or cerebral lesion, but this may not always be so.

There are disturbances of language, articulation and voice that she also has to treat. Ability to understand, express speech and articulate must be tested, assessing tongue and lip movements.

Dysarthria is a neuromuscular problem which causes slurred, weak articulating sounds, sometimes with nasal speech. Usually the meaning of the words is quite clear, but it is the production that is not.

Aphasia is less common than dysarthria and there are two main types. Motor aphasia is when the patient fails to put his thoughts into recognizable words, but can understand all that is said to him. The nurse must never make the unfortunate mistake of talking about the patient in front of him, assuming that he cannot comprehend what is said because he is unable to communicate correctly. Sensory aphasia is when the patient cannot understand the words spoken to him, and means that there is great difficulty in any form of communication.

All the treatment required has to be tailor-made for the patient by the speech therapist, and the nurses must be aware of the lines of treatment, so that they can continue to help the patients in the ward, during their everyday duties of feeding, dressing and bathing them. It is a very individual form of treatment and therefore very time-consuming.

Group therapy for the speech handicapped should be encouraged as this method is of proved psychological as well as clinical benefit.

Rehabilitation of the Elderly Amputee

This is commonly undertaken these days in the geriatric unit and specialized care before and after surgery will ensure good results.

Preoperatively the patient's physical condition will be assessed, especially his cardiovascular and respiratory systems.

The patient must also receive good psychological preparation, a thorough explanation being given to both the patient and the relatives. It may often help if the patient can be visited by a previous amputee who is now home and independent. However, on no account should false hopes be raised.

The patient may have to be transferred to a surgical ward for the actual operation and the first few postoperative days. Pain should be relieved immediately postoperatively and regularly thereafter. The nursing staff should be alert to the fact that the patient may be a little confused for the first 24–48 hours after operation.

The stump should be well bandaged as this helps to keep a good shape, produce less pain and prevent oedema (Fig. 24). The site of the amputation depends on the cause of the operation and the blood supply to the limb. It is usually easiest to rehabilitate those who have a through-knee amputation. If infection is already present, it may be necessary to perform delayed suturing. The majority of these patients are diabetic and therefore healing is slower and the risk of infection may be greater. Infection can lead to oedema, haematoma and osteomyelitis. It is also important for future limb fitting that there is a viable stump flap. Exercises should be given at once after operation, with extension of the limb and prone-lying to prevent flexion. Arm muscles may be improved by the use of a monkey chain and pole.

The patient should be up in a chair as soon as possible and into a wheelchair within a week of surgery. He should be hopping with a walking frame fairly quickly. Provided the stump heals without delay, the patient may visit the limb-fitting centre for the first fitting 2 weeks after surgery and have the limb 2 weeks after that. Depending upon the centre, the patient may have a leg immediately, or may first have a pylon and then a leg. Depending also on the patient's capabilities, the physician in charge of the case may feel that he is not

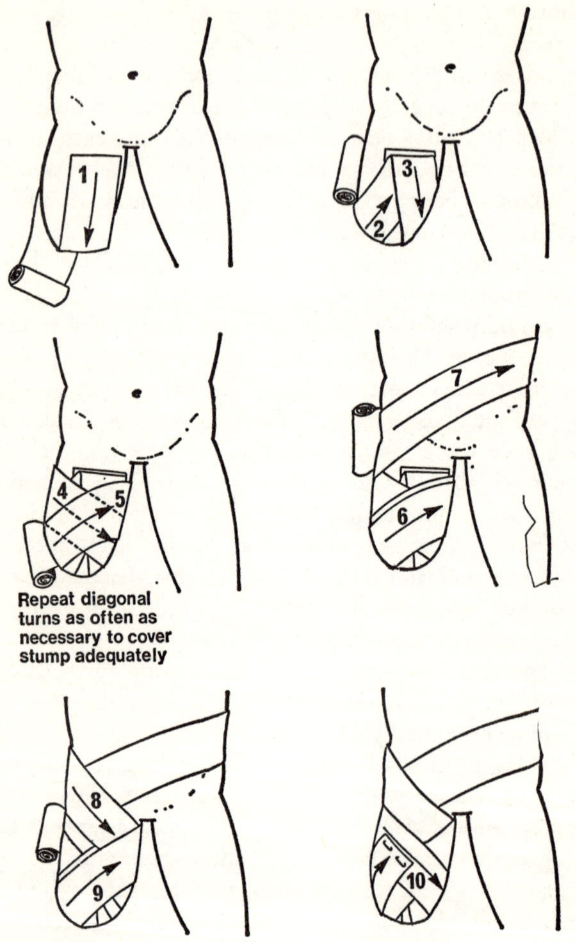

FIG. 24. The method of bandaging a lower limb amputation stump.

fit to graduate from pylon to leg and that the change is not beneficial to the patient.

Case history Miss M., aged 76 years, was admitted from home with gangrene of the right foot. She was an old patient of the geriatric unit with diabetes well controlled by 250 mg of chlorpropamide daily. She had been discharged from the out-patient clinic and was being cared for by her general practitioner. She had had a recent episode of diarrhoëa and vomiting and had collapsed on the floor, where she lay for some hours before a neighbour found her. She was immediately admitted to hospital where intravenous fluids were commenced to correct her dehydration. She was found to have a large gangrenous area on her right heel. Despite conservative treatment the heel failed to improve and Miss M. was given large doses of antibiotics and her insulin was increased to control the rise in blood sugar. The advice of the surgeon was sought and he recommended a through-knee amputation of the right leg. This was carefully explained to Miss M. who accepted the situation quite calmly and signed her consent form. Her brother was also informed. Miss M. was visited by the anaesthetist who found her fit for operation and she was transferred to the surgical ward the night before operation and the amputation was performed the following morning. Post-operative pain was controlled by injection of 50 mg pethidine 4–6 hourly initially and then 2 tablets of Panadol (paracetamol) when necessary. The drain was removed after 48 hours and Miss M. was transferred back to the geriatric unit. She made excellent progress, the stump healed well and sutures were removed after 14 days. A firm bandage was applied 2 or 3 times daily. Miss M. made her first visit to the limb-fitting centre 3 weeks after operation and 10 weeks after operation was walking with a prosthesis. She was discharged to a convalescent home with a view to returning to live alone after a month there.

Some patients who are not well orientated and who may have suffered some residual damage from the anaesthetic, may not benefit at all from a prosthesis, and may well do better to learn to transfer from chair to bed, lavatory, etc. with one leg and rely upon a self-propelling wheelchair for further transport.

Mental Rehabilitation

It has already been emphasized that mental activities are as important as physical exercise and training. Group therapy in the rehabilitation unit instils the will to improve, and also prepares the patient to accept his degree of disability. A short period during the afternoon may be devoted to group therapy and must be carefully organized by the nursing staff, occupational therapists, well supervised voluntary workers or a youth club. Communal activities such as card games, dominoes, bingo, music and movement, frieze work or even folding plastic bags may be enjoyed, and occasionally viewing a few carefully selected slides. In the female ward hairdressing sessions and manicures may be appreciated too.

However, perhaps the best therapy is the happy home life to which the patient is anxious to return. This may be maintained in hospital if visiting is unrestricted and the nursing staff encourage the relatives to visit whenever possible and to help as much as they like and feel able. The help, however, must be constant and not overprotective, as this is sometimes the cause of the patient's being in hospital initially. The unit must not become isolated and outside visits should be arranged whenever practical and possible.

9 Mental Disease in the Elderly

While working within the geriatric unit the nurse will have to deal with the confused patient. States of confusion, some more acute than others, are constantly encountered among the elderly. In addition there are certain degenerative diseases which cause mental disability of various kinds, and a brief description of the more important of these will be given.

Many natural changes occur in the brain during the course of growing old and these include failure of memory, so that incidents which happened many years ago are much clearer than those that occurred quite recently. The elderly person may also experience difficulty with the interpretation of stimuli; therefore bowel and bladder control may become impaired and reactions to taste, smell and pain may be dulled. As we grow older, we find it harder to adapt to new situations; thus change of environment and admission to hospital may have an adverse effect on the elderly, which some take longer to overcome than others. There may also be instability of mental function and a weakening of emotional control whereby the patient may more easily be reduced to tears.

At present 1 in 8 of those in psychiatric hospitals are over 65. During the next decade those over 65 will increase by almost a million and of those half a million will be over 75. By the end of the next decade it is estimated that nearly two-thirds of the patients in mental hospitals may be 65 or more.

So often when caring for the elderly any evidence of confusion or disorientation is quickly and incorrectly referred to as 'senile dementia' and no further attempt is made to investigate the cause or relieve the symptoms.

Confusion

This occurs when the patient loses awareness of himself, finding no significance in time and his surroundings. It is a very common cause of admission to hospital and it is often forgotten that confusion is a symptom underlying a disease and not a disease in itself.

Causes The most common cause is infection, probably with a rise in temperature. Acute chest infections and urinary infections may be accompanied by a period of acute confusion. In fact urinary tract infections may produce few symptoms except for a period of disorientation, and urinary tract infection may not be diagnosed until the result of the examination of the clean urine is received from the pathological laboratory. Once the underlying infection has been treated or treatment has commenced, the confusion will clear.

Cerebral anoxia is another cause of confusion in the elderly. This may be due to an acute disturbance of the blood supply to the brain following a cerebrovascular accident or to failure of the oxygen supply to the brain caused by heart failure, respiratory failure, anaemia or myocardial infarction.

Following surgery cerebral hypoxia (diminished supply of oxygen to the brain) may exist even for a very short period and this can cause damage to the already somewhat precarious brain cells. It may take a patient a little while to compensate for such damage, and thus it is extremely common for a period of confusion to follow surgical intervention. When emergency surgery is performed the nurse must remember that the patient may have been rushed into hospital, into strange surroundings, seen by innumerable different people and taken to theatre all within the space of 24–48 hours, so that he will already be confused on this account.

Disorders of metabolism may also be seen, and confusion may be caused by dehydration, renal failure, diabetes, especially if the patient becomes hypoglycaemic, myxoedema and hypothermia during very cold weather, when the confusion may progress to coma.

Confusion may also occur with deficiency disorders especially with lack of vitamins of the B complex. Once the diagnosis has been established and replacement therapy begun, a rapid improvement will be evident in 10–14 days. The usual treatment is a course of intravenous or intramuscular Parentrovite.

Unfamiliar surroundings may also cause an episode of confusion, especially if the patient is blind or deaf. The elderly person admitted to hospital, who is used to living alone in a small house, will be completely bewildered by the spaciousness of a hospital ward, the innumerable different faces and the continuous activity. Introductions and a guided tour of the ward may help.

Drugs, too, are a common cause of acute confusion in the elderly. If the patient suddenly becomes confused after the start of a new treatment, the nurse must report the fact to the doctor, and the cause must be investigated. If a new drug or drugs have been commenced this should be noted and the dosage reduced if necessary. Frequently the patient has become confused before admission to hospital, and he has been found to be having large doses of drugs which have resulted in the confusional state, e.g. some tranquillizers including the phenothiazine group of drugs, antidepressants especially imipramine and amitriptyline, antiparkinsonian drugs including L-dopa, digoxin, some vasodilators which may improve the blood supply to a specific area by 'stealing' from the rest of the body and sedatives, particularly barbiturates. Great care should be taken at night to give only light sedation and to avoid barbiturates unless the patient has been accustomed to taking them for some time with no ill effects.

The nurse must remember that acute confusion may also occur because the patient has a full bowel or bladder.

Acute confusion may also occur in the patient with an infection superimposed on a chronic disease, resulting in a chronic shortage of oxygen supply to the brain, for instance in chronic heart disease, chronic lung disease and narrowing of the arteries by atheroma or blockage.

All these causes may result in delirium with lack of awareness of events around the patient, illusions and hallucinations which may become more marked at night. The less severe confusional state may last for some weeks even months.

Treatment In view of the many possible causes of confusional states in the elderly, the underlying cause must be discovered before a course of treatment is initiated. When treatment is begun it may be helpful to add vitamin supplements, given by intravenous or intramuscular routes.

The nurse must bear in mind the typical picture of the old man admitted to hospital and put to bed. He suddenly has an urge to micturate and tries to get out of bed. He wanders down the ward, is immediately put back to bed, cot sides are erected and he is heavily sedated. Thus he awakens in the morning far more confused and disorientated. How much simpler it would have been for the enlightened nurse to have shown the patient the way to the lavatory, then taken him to the kitchen, made a cup of tea and had a chat before taking the old man back to bed.

The elderly population must be kept in touch with reality, given their spectacles and encouraged to read the newspaper. Wearing their own clothes, too, helps them to be aware of themselves and their surroundings. It is important that the nursing staff always address patients by their proper names and not by familiar terms of endearment. Bathrooms and lavatories must be clearly indicated, either with colours or with labels in large lettering. The nurse must be aware of the reason for any disorientation that may occur and be prepared to expect this.

The patient must be allowed to do what he likes provided this is safe, and he must not be forcefully restrained. Oversedation must be avoided; if necessary a little thiordiazine may be given for a few days and usually this will be sufficient.

Relatives must be warned and the reason for the confusion explained, as it may be very distressing for them to arrive and find that their elderly relative does not recognize them or appears to be unaware of his surroundings and the period of time in which he is living.

Chronic Brain Syndrome

This is caused by pathological changes affecting the brain tissue itself, the most common types being arteriosclerotic and senile dementia. Very often these are interrelated in varying degrees.

Arteriosclerotic dementia is caused by brain cell atrophy, secondary to arteriosclerosis and a diminishing blood supply. Blood vessels become inelastic, irregular, thickened and narrowed, thus diminishing the flow of blood, and this occurs as a result of ageing alone or because of raised blood pressure and also through dietetic factors. The result is a general dementia with loss of specific brain functions such as speech, voluntary movements of the limbs or an appreciation of sensations.

Senile dementia is caused by brain cell atrophy accompanied by unique microscopic changes, the cause of which is unknown. The patient is unable to remember recent events and suffers from disorientation of time, place and person. He will have a labile (unstable) emotional state. His personal habits become neglectful and clothes become dirty and unkempt. The patient becomes incontinent of both urine and faeces and eventually dies from bronchopneumonia. The onset is gradual and irreversible, and in arteriosclerotic dementia added cerebrovascular incidents may occur with transient paralysis and features of parkinsonism. Post mortem examination of the brain shows general shrinking with dilatation of the ventricles, widening of the sulci (furrows or fissures, especially those of the brain) and narrowing of the gyri convolutions of the brain.

Pre-senile Dementias

These may be seen within the geriatric unit, no other suitable accommodation having been found for the patient.

Alzheimer's Disease

This is a disease resulting in premature ageing, personality changes and impaired memory. Eventually the patient is mute or incoherent. The muscles become stiff and walking is difficult, although the patient may be hyperactive. Terminally the patient is confined to bed, severely demented, totally aphasic and incontinent. There is no specific treatment other than good basic nursing care, and death results from bronchopneumonia.

Pick's Disease

This is similar to Alzheimer's disease, but brain cell loss is restricted to frontal and temporal lobes. The disease is more common in women.

Huntington's Chorea

This is a rare disease, and is a combination of dementia and involuntary movements due to degeneration of the cells of the cortex and extrapyramidal nuclei. It is an inherited disease due to a dominant gene.

Symptoms start between the ages of 30 and 45 years. There is a change of temperament leading to a disintegration of personality, alteration of judgement and memory failure. The limb movements become jerky, irregular and clumsy. As the disease advances walking is impossible and the patient is confined to bed with swallowing impaired. Death usually occurs about 15 years from the onset of symptoms. Some relief occurs from antiparkinsonian agents and tranquillizers.

Dementia Secondary to Infection

With the introduction of penicillin, the treatment of syphilis was radically changed and it is now a curable disease. It can be treated even in the tertiary stage and these syphilitic conditions described are much more rarely seen.

In *cerebrovascular syphilis* damage is limited to the tissues covering the brain, meninges and blood vessels supplying it. The membranes become thickened and the blood vessels narrowed. Symptoms resemble those of arteriosclerotic dementia. In *tabes dorsalis*, damage is limited to the posterior tracts of the spinal cord, which causes impairment of the patient's ability to recognize where his limbs are in space. This results in difficulty in walking. *General paralysis of the insane* develops many years later with mental or physical disorders. Physical disorders include disturbances of speech with slurring of the words. In 50% of the patients, the pupils no longer constrict or dilate but respond only to accommodation.

Multiple Cerebrovascular Accidents and Hemiplegia

These occur generally in patients who are hypertensive and may have been so for some time. Progress is slow, the patient suffers from minor strokes, transient loss of consciousness, fits, falls for no obvious reason and periods of weakness or parasthesia. There are changes of behaviour and mentality. The patient becomes restless, bad-tempered and inconsiderate and personal cleanliness deteriorates markedly. Eventually signs of dementia develop and the disease is progressive and irreversible.

Cerebral Neoplasm

This causes destruction of the surrounding brain cells and irritation of the cells through pressure on them. There is obstruction of the free flow of the cerebrospinal fluid through the ventricles and around the brain. Signs are headaches, giddiness, vomiting, slow pulse and papilloedema, which is caused by obstruction to the venous return from the retina by raised intercranial pressure, causing swelling of the optic discs. Fits occur, with progressive dementia and focal neurological signs. Tumours arising in the frontal lobes are particularly likely to produce personality changes and progressive dementia.

Anaemia

Anaemia superimposed upon an already precarious, but stable, mental state may have disastrous effects. It may increase depression and confusion and aggravate the dementia. Once the cause has been discovered, and replacement therapy begun, the patient should show signs of improvement.

Functional Disorders

Anxiety State

This may show itself first in the elderly patient, but has usually occurred earlier in the patient's life and is not a new manifestation. The patient is usually overanxious about his illness (real or imagined), and subsequent treatment, and this may result in childish behaviour and even incontinence. There may be depression, loss of appetite, preoccupation with bodily function, eventually the patient believing that no part of the body functions as it should.

Case history One elderly lady admitted to hospital with severe bronchopneumonia had had a mild anxiety state for some time. Recently she had lost her husband, son and brother all within the space of 6 months and this had not helped her condition. She rapidly recovered from the bronchopneumonia, but took some time to rehabilitate and become independent again. She had a slight tremor and profuse sweating at times. Her bowels caused her considerable agitation, as they acted infrequently and only with aid. Despite the stools being very soft and the rectum being loaded, she was unable to evacuate this easily. She became more and more agitated, dwelling continuously on the number of days she had been unable to pass a stool. Eventually with the use of fairly strong aperients and a calm attitude on behalf of all the staff, the situation was resolved.

Depression

This is common in the elderly, but often tends not to be diagnosed as the elderly may have a morbid outlook on life. Many patients are loath to admit that they are depressed. Causes are deafness, blindness, pain, immobility, loss of taste, poverty and, perhaps most commonly, bereavement.

There must be a differential diagnosis between myxoedema and depression. There may be impairment of the memory confused with presenile dementia, the patient may become mentally confused or even psychotic in behaviour, this being known as myxoedema madness. Other signs and symptoms of myxoedema will be present.

Reactive or exogenous depression There are numerous reasons for this condition especially among patients admitted to hospital. If they live alone they may be concerned as to whether they will be able to return home and manage alone again. They become depressed at the thought of having to give up their home and independence, and perhaps live in a home or residential accommodation organized by the council. Some may feel rejected by their relatives, life may have been difficult at home and the family may have become resentful of their elderly relative living with them. The old person may realize this and become depressed at feeling a burden. Others may worry at the thought of having to return home to relatives whom they think cannot manage, but become depressed at the thought of having to spend the rest of their life in hospital or a home.

Endogenous depression This has usually begun in earlier life and persists into old age. The patients partake in few activities, everything is too much effort. They dislike food and suffer from lack of concentration. They experience delusions of guilt, poverty, hypochondria and nihilistic delusions. They may feel that part of their body is dead. These people often do better if treated at home, but not if they are suicidal or if the home environment is unsuitable.

There is a high rate of suicides in the elderly, especially amongst men, many of whom suffer from the endogenous type of depression. Contributory factors include loneliness, bereavement and physical illness. Ill-planned retirement may have some link with the higher rate among men. All threats should be taken seriously and many may need a period of hospitalization.

Signs These may include agitation, sleeplessness with wandering at night, aimless wandering during the day, loss of appetite resulting in nutritional deficiencies and malnutrition, constipation, loss of interest in self and surroundings with some confusion, neglect of home and person and failure to respond to approaches or to answer questions. These people are very reluctant to be admitted to hospital.

Treatment Treatment may be by psychotrophic drugs such as imipramine or by a course of electroconvulsive therapy.

Much will depend upon the staff of the ward, and the atmosphere within the ward. The degree of social contact will also depend upon this and the policy of the ward, and the attitude towards social activities. The social worker can play an active part here, just by listening to the patient's worries or by helping to organize some form of social diversion.

Bereavement Syndrome

Severe depression may occur in the elderly who have lost a close friend or relative on whom they are dependent, particularly a spouse. It usually occurs in those who already have a tendency to depression. The episode of depression may last for several weeks or even months, but generally clears with help from social workers, clergy, therapists and nurses when the patient is in hospital.

Case History Mrs B. was admitted from home having lost her husband 6 weeks previously. She was a pleasant lady who had a history of ischaemic heart disease for several years, and mild depression at times. On the death of her husband she became acutely depressed and was now quite unable to cope alone. Initially on admission to the ward, she was quite cheerful and able, but gradually reverted to her original state of acute depression. She was visited by a psychiatrist and treatment with antidepressant drugs was commenced. Improvement became quite marked and soon she was considered fit to return home. At the mention of this she deteriorated rapidly. As she had been well able to cope at home prior to her husband's death it was decided to send her home to see how she would manage having given her maximum support and having alerted the social services and the psychiatrist. Unfortunately the patient declined rapidly at home, and was admitted to a psychiatric hospital for another period of treatment.

Paraphrenia

This is a form of schizophrenia occurring in the elderly, especially spinsters living alone, and rather isolated. They have feelings of being spied upon, and that their neighbours may be transmitting rays across to them causing some harm. There are known cases of houses being boarded up with newspapers against this evil, so that the rays are not able to get through. Such patients are generally difficult to control.

Mania and hypomania

These patients are cheerful and confident. They are supremely fit and able, and become restless and noisy if not treated. Whilst in their manic state, food and drink may be omitted and they may feel they are being poisoned, and they may become more preoccupied with the cause of the manic state. Eventually if no treatment is given, they become exhausted, suffering from dehydration and malnutrition. They may be treated with parenteral tranquillizers such as haloperidol.

General Principles of Treatment

Admission to hospital should be avoided whenever possible as change of surroundings or environment can be disastrous to a slightly demented old person. These people manage well at home but become severely disabled if removed from their familiar surroundings, and tend to become long-stay patients. They should be supported at home for as long as possible. Every area should have community-orientated services with meals-on-wheels and home helps. Home laundry, home chiropody and day hospital care should be available if necessary.

If hospital admission is necessary, 5 % of these patients may go into general beds as they have some underlying physical disease. It is extremely important that the patient is kept occupied and up-to-date. Group activities should be arranged, and the nursing staff should be free to accompany the patient. Boredom must be avoided, and the patient should be placed so that he can see what is going on in the ward and around him. These patients tend to become anxious if they are put in the middle of the room or near a wall.

The nurse should ensure that the patient is wearing spectacles if necessary, and encourage him to read the newspaper, thus keeping in touch with reality. These patients may be helped by having various rooms, e.g. bathroom and lavatory, identified by different coloured doors. They should be supervised without restraint and cot sides should be avoided as they may only increase the agitation.

The elderly patient suffering from mental disorder is particularly sensitive to disapproval or affection and touch is important when there is mental impairment. In all cases it is extremely important to give back their self-respect and where possible to allow patients to have a say in their future.

It may be helpful to give the patient a drug which will

improve the brain metabolism which has been damaged by lack of oxygen, e.g. Cyclospasmol, Lucidril, Praxilene, Hydergine. It helps the patient to become more aware of his bowel and bladder needs and generally more aware of his surroundings.

Assessment and improvement may be aided with the use of memory and concentration tests used before and after a period of treatment.

For those who are able to be maintained in the community, day hospital facilities should be available in either the general or the psychiatric hospital. The day should be well organized with a friendly greeting on arrival and time over coffee to chat to the staff. Physical and mental stimulation must be included, familiar songs may be sung and even dancing may be enjoyed.

Personal care should be attended to. Feeding may require assistance and assessment. Daily baths may be given and hair-dressing, make-up and manicure all provide a boost to the patient's morale. Chiropody may be provided also, and the patient will be able to attend the physiotherapy department if necessary. A doctor will be in attendance so that medical needs may be assessed, as well as the conditions of ears, eyes, feet, bladder and bowels.

All these services may help the patient to be maintained at home alone or with his family for some time, rather than being admitted to hospital which will inevitably result in a deterioration in general orientation and mental disturbance.

10 Care of the Long-stay Patient and the Dying

The Long-stay Patient

The long-stay patient is seen as a medical and/or social failure, and therefore could be termed the end of the line in nursing and geriatrics. The very existence of such patients constitutes a problem of considerable magnitude. Caring for this category of patient is arduous, monotonous and fraught with difficulties. It is discouraging for the nursing staff to see little return for their labours. There is a greater incidence of women than of men, partly because the expectation of life for women is greater than for men (74·7 years compared to 68·6 years) (Registrar General 1966), and because women survive longer living with their disabilities, whereas men tend not to survive very long once they fall ill. If her husband has died previously, there is often no one left to look after the wife when she becomes ill and old. In the unit where the author works the average length of stay is from 1 to 2 years and may be over 5 years. There is need for frequent reassessment, as some patients continue to improve in the slow tempo of the long-stay wards. Doctors visit to treat specific medical illness and review some patients who might profit from a further period on the rehabilitation ward.

The numbers of long-stay patients are increasing steadily due to the considerable increase in the proportion of older elderly.

The long-stay wards and annexes are the successors of the chronic sick wards, in that they house and nurse patients who make little or no progress. Because of progressive physical or mental disability and failure to respond to treatment or remedial therapy, the patients require indefinite nursing with intermittent medical attention. The patients build up resistance to further physical onslaughts and infection, and as a result they may live in this state for many years.

The siting of the ward is important and not always ideal. Many long-stay units are found in old workhouses, often in an isolated part of the town and in rather dreary surroundings. The elderly still remember the time when old people were taken into custodial care in overcrowded and spartan conditions. Patients need to be within easy reach of visitors and pleasant surroundings so that they may sit outside in the summer and enjoy gardens and grounds wherever possible. It is also therapeutic for patients to see some activity in the outside world, such as traffic and people passing by, as they should not feel isolated from the community. Although not requiring all the facilities of a district general hospital, the long-stay unit does require the services of the physiotherapy and occupational therapy units. It is therefore best sited away from the general hospital in annexes, where the accent is on a more homely atmosphere, slower tempo and less rigid ward routine.

Nursing within this unit is of a specialized nature and not suitable for all nurses. Some prefer to nurse patients where more positive treatment is possible and there is a much quicker turnover of patients within the ward. Others feel they have something to offer in this field and enjoy the constant contact with the same patients. It is extremely important to maintain a high morale among the staff and this can only be done by developing a good team spirit, so that all are working together and helping to overcome the many problems and difficulties encountered in these wards. Not only must the nurses form a team, but doctors, physiotherapists, occupational therapists, social workers and voluntary workers must also give their help and support. Nurses are required to combine basic nursing skills with traditional courtesy, kindness and sense of duty. The permanent staff caring for long-stay patients and those with antisocial and unpleasant tendencies calls for nurses older in experience and emotionally more mature and stable. However, student and pupil nurses gaining geriatric experience should be encouraged to work on these wards for a limited period of time, as old people like to see the young about them and the generations get on well together.

The ward is the patient's home, so the atmosphere must be somewhat different to that of the busy general ward and the patients should be surrounded by their personal possessions, ornaments and photographs. Sometimes it is possible for them to have their own chair, if it is suitable, in the ward. The nurse should try to investigate the patient's past, his previous occupation, and what happened to his family, so that she can visualize the patient as he was when he was fit and well, and also show a constructive interest in the patient's present affairs. Perhaps the patient has some interesting hobbies and these could be renewed and pursued in hospital. It is surprising how many patients can still perform simple jobs and make themselves useful despite a physical or mental handicap. It is also very important to maintain their self-respect and, if possible, make the patients feel they are useful and have a purpose in life.

The patients should be dressed every day, whenever possible, and should wear their own clothes. Many of these patients have no suitable clothes and it may be necessary to acquire some for them. Nowadays, with Crimplene dresses readily available, there is no excuse for an old lady to wear old woollen cast-offs which do not fit. Wearing their own clothes gives patients an identity and pride in their appearance. They should also be encouraged to wear good shoes; no one can attempt to walk successfully if they only wear bedroom slippers, giving no support to the feet. Clothes for the disabled are now readily available and can usually be acquired on contract through the hospital suppliers. There are a variety of attractively designed and coloured dresses specifically for the disabled and incontinent. For ladies there are short vests, split dresses and skirts in Crimplene and similar easily washable non-iron materials which are crease-resistant. Self-support hose remove the necessity for corsets and suspender belts. Of course pants should be worn at all times. For the men there are especially adapted trousers with Velcro fastenings and openings as necessary. There are also especially adapted braces and toe-less socks, sweaters of various descriptions and coats split down the middle with a Velcro fastening for the immobile patient. For the bedridden patient there are now a variety of nightdresses which are easy to put on, but do not have an institutional look. Laundering of the patients' own clothing often proves difficult. Ideally, but not often practically, it is best if the visitors can assist in this field. However, failing this, the hospital laundry may be helpful and some units are lucky enough to have a launderette attached to the day hospital. Marking poses another problem and is unfortunately essential to prevent loss of valuable clothing. It is, however, a job that can be undertaken by visitors or voluntary workers.

Incontinence is also a problem often encountered in the long stay ward and must be treated optimistically with a realistic outlook by the staff. If all other methods fail, there should be no reservations in resorting to a catheter and leg bag during the day and free drainage at night. It is also possible to have the tubing of the catheter bag passing through the vest seam and the bag itself contained in a sponge bag. This is more satisfactory than a spigot when the patient is up, as the latter tends to cause more frequent urinary tract infection. Faecal incontinence should rarely occur if the patient's bowel habits are well supervised. Incontinence is discussed in detail in Chapter 5.

The patients must be encouraged to maintain a pride in their appearance, and a regular visit from a hairdresser is a necessity. Nothing is more successful in boosting the morale of the elderly lady than to have her hair permed or set. Similarly the elderly men should have a daily shave and a visit from the barber when necessary. Nails should be kept clean and short. Hearing aids should be kept in good working order, and false teeth should be seen to be comfortable and well-fitting.

Feeding, too, may prove a problem. The patients should be encouraged to feed themselves for as long as possible. There is nothing more degrading and unpleasant than having to be fed by someone else. In order to feed himself comfortably and successfully the patient should be sitting as easily as possible, preferably in a chair, as it is difficult to sit upright in bed, with easy access to the table and tray. Various aids should be available on the ward to help patients with specific disabilities. Hemiplegic patients have difficulty in managing single-handed and may benefit from a plate bunker or bowl produced by Melaware products especially designed for the handicapped and disabled. The Nelson knife may be beneficial in certain cases. Melaware, in their Manoy range of goods, also produce a well-designed cup and various pieces of cutlery which may be of help to those disabled by arthritis or who have Parkinson's disease. These three diseases especially provide many problems for the staff and patients at meal times. Unfortunately some form of bib is often desirable if the patient's clothes are to be kept clean and presentable. Cindico produce a valuable plastic bib with a shelf at the bottom for the really messy eater.

Activities in the long-stay ward should be so designed as to stimulate the patients, make them feel useful members of society within their own sphere, and if possible also provide some remedial exercise. These activities are sometimes arranged by the occupational therapists, nurses or again there is a good opening for the right kind of voluntary worker. Patients may be able to knit or sew without difficulty and could make clothes or blankets for a charitable organization. Some may still enjoy cooking and could bake a cake for the ward tea, or may be able to help with the washing up at meal times. If the patient is able, she should be encouraged to make her own bed with the help of the nurse. Group activities in the form of music and movement, singing or frieze work are often enjoyed and may be beneficial. Outings are particularly necessary as many of the patients have not seen the outside world for some time, and it is amazing what stimulation a short drive can produce. In some areas Age Concern or Toc H can arrange this. Also shopping expeditions or a visit to the local cinema, if easily accessible, are much enjoyed. Films organized at regular intervals by travel clubs, epic film societies and local film clubs are much appreciated provided the patients do not have to sit for too long.

A good liaison should be kept with the chaplains of the various denominations as the patients appreciate talks with them. Arrangements should be made for patients to attend chapel services, or for services to be held in the ward. Sometimes it is possible for them to attend a local church and to be made to feel a member of the community. Here again there is a helpful rôle for the voluntary worker or a local church youth group.

If the long-stay wards are housed within the unit, it may be possible for the staff and patients to join in communal activities; an occasional party is very popular and a source of amusement. To see new faces is always stimulating and refreshing. The library should visit the ward at least once a week, and the mobile shop should call daily, and provide newspapers, sweets, writing paper and toilet articles.

Nurses must have time to sit and talk to their patients, as so often the patient may lose the art of communication. Similarly the patients should be grouped in the day room with those of similar outlook and interests. The severely confused should be separated from the more rational patients. There can be nothing more aggravating or soul-destroying than having to sit day by day with those patients with whom one has nothing in common. It requires imagination and initiative by the nurses to group them correctly.

It is important to have open visiting; then relatives and friends may be involved with the patient's care wherever possible, even if it is only occasionally helping the patient to feed. This is one of the advantages in having the long-stay annexe in the community it serves, rather than isolated many miles away.

Younger Chronic Sick

This unfortunate group of people is still found on the long-stay geriatric wards, although adequate provision is now made for some of them in units of their own; unfortunately these are often far away from their own homes.

In 1970 the Chronically Sick and Disabled Persons Act was passed and ensured that every local authority was aware of the numbers and needs of the disabled living in its area who are registered. The local authority should help the disabled and provide facilities to enable them to live at home for as long as possible, if necessary providing special accommodation. When this proves no longer possible or practicable, hospitals must do all they can to ensure that those under 65 are not cared for in wards used for the care of the elderly infirm.

The problems of these younger chronic sick are threefold:

physical, psychological and social. Those who find themselves in these units are normally those patients suffering from medical, surgical or neurological conditions, e.g. chronic pulmonary, cardiac or renal conditions, poliomyelitis, muscular dystrophy, multiple sclerosis and severe arthritis.

These patients naturally require special units adapted for their care, with physiotherapy and occupational therapy near at hand. They need to maintain their independence wherever possible and to have every facility for occupation and entertainment available. For them particularly the hospital becomes their home, therefore privacy should be given them wherever possible, with small rooms available for those who prefer them. Activities need to be therapeutic, and some patients may be able to follow in some way their previous hobbies or professions. Frequent outings and entertainments must be organized.

This type of nursing requires the development of certain skills by the nurse. Great patience is required together with imagination and a sense of humour. The relatives need much support and help and will be greatly assisted by the help and advice of the social worker. The relatives should be encouraged to visit as often as possible and to partake in the life of the ward and the patient.

Care of the Dying

Not a lot is written on this subject, nor is much taught to nurses and doctors, but it is a very important aspect of their work, especially in the geriatric unit. Although the accent is on a positive, progressive approach and on rehabilitation, statistics show that in the acute assessment ward alone 30% of the patients die within the first few weeks of admission, so this aspect of nursing must be met daily and much can be learnt and taught in this sphere.

Ideally most elderly patients should die at home in surroundings familiar to them and with those they love around them. No patient should be brought into hospital just to die, but many die there having failed to respond to treatment, or having ended their lives in the long-stay ward. People prefer to die in their own homes, and the difficulty arises when they can no longer be nursed there and have to come into hospital to receive the adequate basic care required. Services in the community are far from adequate as yet, although laundry services for the incontinent patient and various aids are available from some local authorities. Night attendance is difficult to obtain; the night and day attendance allowance is difficult to acquire as the conditions for eligibility are severe, and the family may suffer from financial hardship.

The nurse is required to give total care to these patients, not only physical but also mental care. The majority of patients need frequent attention—daily bath, 2-hourly care of pressure areas and mouth. The patients are particularly prone to pressure sores and these must be prevented as they are only a cause of further pain and discomfort. A dry mouth and dehydration must be prevented also. Frequent cleaning with glycerine and thymol or glycerine and borax help to keep the mouth fresh. Encouraging frequent small refreshing drinks and occasionally sucking ice cubes all help. Dry lips respond well to petroleum jelly or Nivea cream.

Various discomforts can be relieved by good nursing. Many patients suffer from breathlessness and this can be relieved by good positioning, nursing them either upright in bed with their pillows placed in an 'armchair' or in a chair so that they can remain comfortably upright; the Buxton chair is very useful here. Many patients with terminal disease suffer from nausea and vomiting, which can be most distressing. The patient should be nursed in bed if this is more comfortable for him; suitable and acceptable drinks should be given; again ice may be sucked as this keeps the mouth fresh and moist. Occasionally anti-emetic drugs need to be given either orally or by injection, and the nurse should see that such a drug is given a short while before the meal. The patient may suffer from anorexia, and a little sherry before meals may help to overcome this and make the food more palatable. A little food, well presented, may tempt the patient to eat a little. Bowels and bladder will also need routine care. If the patient becomes incontinent of urine, there are no contraindications to catheterization for the terminally ill, and this may relieve restlessness and discomfort from an overdistended bladder or a perpetually wet bed. Bowels should be observed and relieved where necessary with an enema or glycerine suppositories. A gentle laxative such as Senokot or Dorbanex may prove helpful, but it must be remembered that if the patient is taking very little solid food, he is unlikely to have a regular bowel action.

The relief of pain for the dying patient is a difficult aspect of their care, but nevertheless a very important one. Minor aches and mild pain can be relieved with aspirin, codeine or paracetamol given regularly, but severe pain needs the use of opiates, particularly heroin. It is often beneficial to give chlorpromazine combined with a pain-relieving drug. Analgesics should be given regularly in a sufficient dosage to relieve pain and assure the patient that the pain is well controlled. So often the nurse waits to be told that the patient has pain before administering the analgesia instead of giving a regular dosage so that no pain is experienced There are various mixtures commonly used for the terminally ill, which contain heroin and/or morphine, cocaine, alcohol and an acceptable flavouring, which, given orally, will successfully relieve pain and give the patient a sense of well being.

There may be insomnia, and the nurse should attend to the simple necessities of the patient before resorting to sedatives.

The nurse should ensure that the patient is comfortable, that the bladder and bowels are not full, that the patient is well positioned and warm enough. Many patients suffer from poor peripheral circulation, and require bedsocks or a hot-water bottle, provided it is not filled with boiling water, and is adequately protected to avoid burns. An additional bed jacket, mittens or a soft extra blanket may all be helpful. A warm soothing drink such as brandy and milk may be welcomed. Finally, any pain present must obviously be relieved, and if all else fails, a mild sedative or hypnotic may be used, such as chloral or nitrazepam.

The loneliness of the dying patient is often severe. The nursing staff tend to avoid these patients through fear and anxiety that they may be asked questions they cannot answer. The patients must have confidence in those caring for them and time must be given to them to relate their symptoms even if they are already known, and the nurse must be prepared to spend time just listening to their fears and anxieties. So often, no advice or help is sought from the nurse, only a sympathetic ear. At least 25 % of patients know that they are dying, and for the elderly it may be a relief from long suffering, loneliness and the discomfort of later life. The majority of elderly patients have a different approach to death from that of the younger patient. The truth may have dawned on them without their being told, and they may not wish to discuss this. The art of listening is something to be learnt by all those who work in this field.

On the whole, the patients are anxious only when they do not know their future, but are at peace when they know that death is near. Occasionally tranquillizers may be needed to help to relieve anxiety. When death is inevitable, the patient should be allowed to die in peace, unencumbered by useless apparatus. Religious beliefs must be respected and the help of the clergy should be sought at an early stage. The patient's belief is obviously relevant when considering death and those with a faith die with less anxiety or apprehension. Loneliness too may be due to lack of visitors, who hesitate to visit the dying. Relatives should be encouraged to visit wherever possible and should be helped and supported by all the staff, not only the nurses but also the social workers. The relatives too must have confidence in those who are caring for their relative. Many elderly spouses will need much support and comfort after the death of a husband or wife. This support should be given by the social worker, family doctor and health visitor. The nurse should find out at an early stage whether the relative wishes to be called at night should the patient deteriorate or die. When the patient has died, discretion should be exercised in informing the relatives. If they live alone, it may be done through the police, family doctor or a close friend. Some relatives like to view the patient after death, and this may be arranged either in the mortuary chapel or the chapel of the funeral director.

Last Offices

When the patient has died, the doctor should be notified immediately and will confirm that death has actually taken place. The nurse should then lay the patient flat, straighten all the limbs, clean the mouth and position the false teeth, bind the jaw, close the eyes with damp cotton wool and cover the patient with a sheet having stripped the rest of the bed of bedding. All pillows, air rings, etc. should be removed, and any tubes should also be removed except in exceptional circumstances. The patient may then be left for up to one hour.

The final care of the patient should be administered by two nurses, one of whom should be senior and experienced in this work. The bed should be well screened off so that no one can possibly see the patient. The nurse will wash the patient, plugging the rectum, and the vagina in the female patient, and placing sleek or waterproof plaster over any open sores. The body is dressed in a suitable gown and clearly labelled, before being placed in a mortuary sheet and removed to the mortuary. All the patient's possessions should be listed and packed up, to be stored safely, preferably in the administrative offices. Valuables should be checked and locked away to await collection by the relatives.

The dignity of the patient should be preserved at all times.

11 Social Care

Since as early as 1536 there has been legislation to give help to the 'poor, impotent, lame, feeble, sick and diseased persons' under the old Poor Laws. Such help was often given grudgingly and the receipt of it implied a social stigma. The passing of the National Assistance Act 1948, which has been brought up to date by the Chronically Sick and Disabled Persons Act 1970, lays a duty on local authorities to provide such help as will be discussed in this chapter and seeks to dispel the idea that assistance is 'charity'. However this idea does persist in the minds of many of the elderly who remember the old days of the workhouses.

Today the major duty of providing help for the disabled is undertaken by the State, but there is a big role for voluntary bodies, working with the statutory bodies. Over one million elderly in this country live alone, and of these more than 5% are both alone and unable to care for themselves adequately. Since the passing of the Chronically Sick and Disabled Persons Act in 1970, local authorities are required to keep a register of disabled persons in their areas and by far the largest group of blind, deaf and otherwise handicapped persons are 65 years of age and over.

The first aim of those concerned with the welfare of the elderly is to keep them as fit as possible, and since old people need a sense of belonging, enable them to live in their own homes, either alone or with their families. Many are able to continue to lead the kind of life they have always enjoyed, supported by family and friends, and may never require the services of the local authority. However from the age of 80 years onwards the elderly are more frail and more prone to sickness so that there is a greater likelihood that help may be needed.

Statutory Bodies

In order to understand what help can be provided and how it may be obtained, it is necessary to consider briefly the reorganized National Health Service and the Social Services departments of the local authorities. Since April 1974 the NHS has expanded to include such domiciliary workers as home nurses and health visitors who were formerly employed by the local authorities; at the same time the social services departments of the local authorities have included in their teams of social workers those who work within the hospitals, formerly known as medical social workers. These two services must not only work closely together themselves but must also maintain cooperation with the family practitioner service. The general practitioner may often be the first point of contact with the elderly in need of help and in many areas home nurses, health visitors and even social workers are attached to general practices. The home nurse will carry out any necessary practical nursing procedures. The health visitor will visit those elderly persons referred to her by the general practitioner; ideally she would visit all old people on the practice list, but because of the size of her case load and the diversity of her work it is usually possible to keep only those known to be at risk under regular supervision. In some areas a health visitor may be attached to a geriatric unit and will visit the patient before his admission to hospital, during his stay there and after his discharge. Again, in some areas health visitors or registered nurses are employed to look after geriatric patients only, the accent being on preventive medicine.

The care and welfare of the elderly is also one of the responsibilities of the social services departments of local

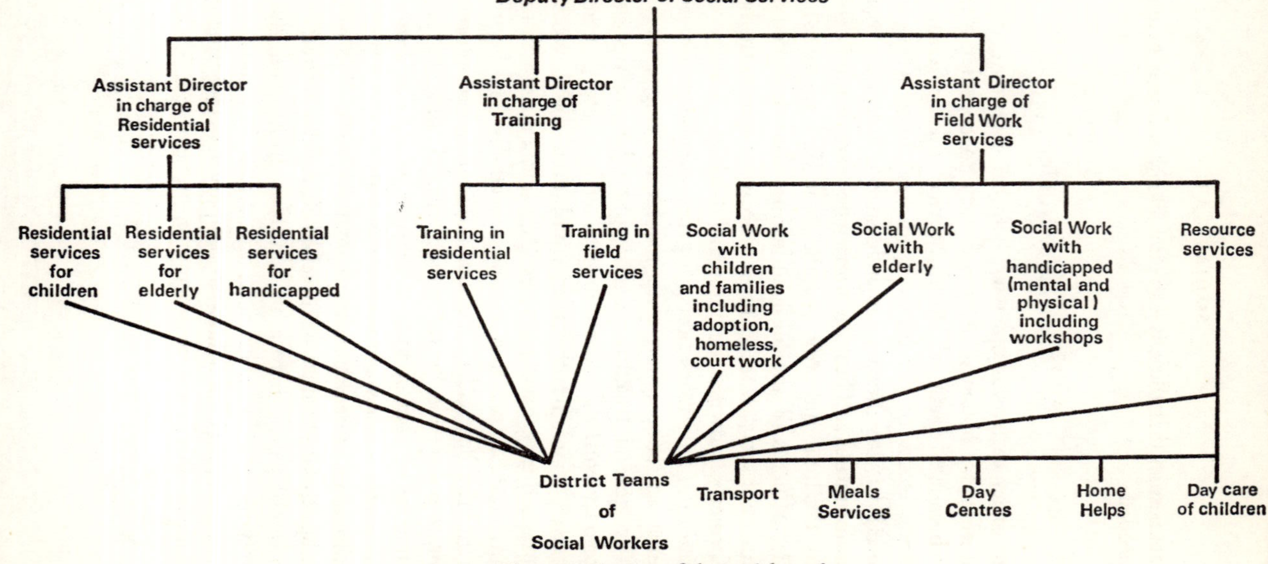

FIG. 25. The organisation of the social services.

authorities. Their main aim again is preventive, and to this end they are empowered to provide a number of services, including home helps who will carry out household cleaning for the elderly, cook a meal where necessary and do essential shopping; the 'meals-on-wheels' service (carried out either by the local authority itself or by the Women's Royal Voluntary Service for the local authority); transport; 'good neighbour' schemes in which a neighbour will help an elderly person living near by; luncheon clubs; and other services. For some of the services provided by the local authority, for example the provision of home help, a charge is made. However the contribution asked for will depend on the means of the individual; those living on retirement pensions or supplementary pensions are exempt from payment altogether.

It must be emphasized that, while the local authority has a statutory duty to care for the elderly, the actual services which each authority is able to provide depend upon the facilities which are available and therefore these may vary greatly from area to area. In all areas there are social workers who visit the elderly and help them with any problems.

Housing of the elderly is obviously of great importance. Each local authority provides various types of accommodation ranging from independent flatlets to groups of flatlets in which there is a warden to keep an eye on the elderly and summon help when necessary, to residential accommodation. In this latter are housed old people who are able to get up, dress (although perhaps needing assistance), have a reasonable degree of mobility and eat a meal without help. Those who are too frail to manage these minimum requirements are the responsibility of the National Health Service and may need to be cared for in long-stay hospitals or day hospitals (see Chapters 2 and 12). Housing of the elderly is further discussed on p. 210.

Perhaps the ideal form of housing for the elderly is living

with the family and yet having separate facilities. However, it is not in every family that this can be achieved and many old people are fiercely independent and may refuse to live with the family although there may be an obvious need for them to do so. Many old people still live in grossly inadequate and unsuitable accommodation, presenting a problem which may tax the ingenuity and resources of the social services.

From this review of some of the services that are available to old people from the family practitioner service, the National Health Service and the local authority social services departments it will be seen that to ensure the best that can be done for the old and disabled a high degree of liaison and good will between those helping them is a first priority.

Voluntary Organizations

Since 1940 voluntary services for old people throughout the country have been coordinated and related to statutory services through Age Concern, originally known as the Old People's Welfare Committee, which is represented at regional, county and local level, and is concerned with the care of the elderly in the area. Age Concern aims 'to study the needs of old people and to encourage and promote measures for their well being'. It ensures regular consultation between all bodies and individuals who are able to help to bring adequate welfare service to the elderly, irrespective of their background or income. It aims to provide the more personal services not made available locally by the health or social services, concentrating on providing help, information, advice and encouragement at the right moment. The following services are made available by Age Concern, but not all in every area:

Visiting
Advice and information

- Individual services—shopping, reading aloud, gardening, decorating, escorting, hairdressing
- Day centres, lunch clubs, social clubs
- Laundry
- Chiropody
- Transport by car, wheelchair or special vehicle
- Mobile libraries
- Holidays
- Outings and entertainments
- Housing
- Employment and job finding
- Exhibitions and competitions
- Help in emergencies
- Youth help
- Residential homes and help with accommodation problems
- Aids for the infirm
- Day and night sitter-in services
- Spiritual aspects
- Prevention of accidents
- Provision and repair of radio and television sets

The Council for Social Service also aims to provide services for old people, either directly or through associated groups.

Day centres, social clubs, lunch clubs are all places where the elderly can attend daily, weekly or even bi-weekly, in order to enjoy nourishing food and congenial society. Most towns have a day centre where transport is provided, and the elderly arrive in time for morning coffee and leave after tea. They can have a bath and the hairdresser and chiropodist may attend. Entertainment may be laid on, cards, sewing, knitting and conversation enjoyed and outings organized.

It is important to help the elderly to continue at work for as long as they are willing and able to do so, although it is difficult with the retirement age tending to decrease. Careful planning should be made before retirement. People should be encouraged to remain amongst their friends rather than to isolate themselves in some beautiful area or seaside resort. It may be necessary to move to a more suitable house or flat with easy access and easily managed heating facilities.

The Employment Fellowship is a small charity whose principal object is to encourage and assist in setting up and establishing sheltered workshops for the elderly. Now there are approximately 100 work centres in the United Kingdom occupying some 4000 old-age pensioners.

Task Force, which is a voluntary youth organization with a local authority grant, operates in London, and similar groups, Youth Volunteer Action, etc., operate in the provinces, aiming to help the aged and handicapped. Organized by a paid official, they run schemes, often through schools and youth groups, for visiting the elderly, doing their shopping, decorating the house and gardening. Visits from the young are generally much appreciated by the elderly.

The Women's Royal Voluntary Service provides various services for the elderly. The best known is Meals-on-Wheels, which is subsidized by the local authority and provides an essential service for many elderly people who are unable to cook their own meals. In many towns meals are available 5 days a week, but in rural areas where transport is difficult the service may be provided only once or twice a week. The Women's Royal Voluntary Service also have luncheon clubs for the elderly. Some branches of the service regularly visit the elderly in their own homes.

The local branches of the Red Cross Society also provide some helpful home services including loans of equipment such as commodes, wheelchairs, chairs, beds and walking aids. They may also help with home nursing for limited periods, providing night sitters and transport if required. They will take the elderly to hospital for out-patient appointments, to visit relatives in hospital and even take the housebound for occasional drives.

Financial Assistance

The great majority of the elderly are entitled to a pension. The 1948 National Insurance Act produced a comprehensive system of insurance against loss of income by interruption of earnings. It established an extended system of national insurance, providing payments by way of unemployment benefits, maternity benefits, retirement pensions, widows' benefits, guardians' allowances and death grants. Insured persons qualify for a retirement pension when they reach the minimum pensionable age—65 for men, 60 for women. If retirement is postponed, the pension becomes payable when they give up regular employment and automatically at the age of 70 years. Pensioners receive a pension book containing weekly orders payable at a local post office. Each order is valid for three months. If the elderly person is unable to attend the post office, he may authorize some other person to draw the pension. If the pensioner is admitted to hospital, the pension is reduced after 8 weeks.

Poor law legislation ended in 1948 and was replaced by the National Assistance Act 1948. The National Assistance Board took over the responsibility for meeting the financial needs of persons without resources and those whose resources were insufficient for their needs. In 1966 the Supplementary Benefits Commission was established under the Department of Health and Social Security to award (*a*) supplementary pensions for those persons over pensionable age and (*b*) supplementary allowances for those under pensionable age. A person of pensionable age not in full-time work, has a right to a supplementary pension if his income requirements plus a sum for rent fall below a certain minimum level. To make a claim a book of orders for this supplement is presented at the post office together with the retirement pension book.

In 1970, under the National Insurance (Old Persons and Widows Pensions and Attendance Allowance) Act, people who were over pensionable age in 1948 and were thus excluded from the National Insurance scheme, became entitled to a pension.

Provision for an attendance allowance was made available from 1971 to give financial aid to the disabled living at home under considerable difficulty. Conditions for the payment of allowance are that one of the following medical requirements be satisfied for a period of at least 6 months:

1. The person is so severely disabled physically or mentally that he requires from another person, in connection with his bodily functions, frequent attention during the day and prolonged repeated attention during the night.

2. The person is so severely disabled physically or mentally that he requires continual supervision from another person in order to avoid danger to himself or others.

Residential Accommodation

Many old people who are not able to live alone, *do not* require a hospital bed, but *do* require residential accommodation providing minimal care and attention. Most people decide of their own accord that they want to move into a home and at present there are over half a million old people living in such institutions in this country voluntarily. Under the National Assistance Act 1948, Section 47, certain powers are given to the Community Physician to arrange the removal of persons needing care and attention who suffer grave chronic disease or, being aged and infirm or physically handicapped, live in insanitary conditions and are unable to give themselves, and do not receive, proper care and attention. Application must be made to the magistrates and a limited period in care is applied which may be extended.

The National Health Service Act 1946, the National Assistance Act 1948 and Mental Health Act 1959 stated that local authorities must provide residential accommodation for mentally and physically handicapped people and the elderly. Under Part III of the National Assistance Act, the needs for residential accommodation for the elderly are considered. This is provided by the local authority in homes of their own, or in homes managed by voluntary organizations, or in private homes registered for the purpose; the latter two sorts of home receive some financial aid from the local authority. Under the same act, all private homes for the elderly or disabled must be registered with the local authority so that they can be inspected to see that they are properly equipped and maintained at a reasonable standard. All these homes aim to provide a homely atmosphere and to meet all reasonable requirements of the residents including clothing, extra comforts and services, recreational facilities, books, periodicals, radio and television. Staff provide care and attention and such nursing care as would be given by relatives in their own home, the help of the home nurse may be enlisted. The accommodation is not always ideal as suitable houses are not always available; but now, especially designed homes are being built which are well planned and have appropriate facilities. Finding and keeping suitable staff is often a problem.

All persons provided with residential accommodation must pay. If unable to pay the standard rate, they are assessed according to income, always being allowed to keep some pocket money.

There are many reasons which may lead to a person having to give up his own home life and enter a residential home. Some people feel they can no longer live alone. A large proportion come from homes where they have been living with their families; family conflicts with the younger generation or unpleasant habits make them or the family feel they can cope no longer. The habits and ways of life of the elderly grandparents and the growing up grandchildren are so widely different that it is not often possible for them all to live together in a confined space. Of course, many families do make the effort and it is often entirely successful.

12 Discharge and the Patient's Future

Preparation for Discharge

The aim of the geriatric unit is to make the patient fit and ready for discharge. This is what it is hoped will be achieved by successful treatment and rehabilitation. As always, the whole team is involved, including all those in the community, as careful preparation for discharge is always required. A suitable day will be selected well in advance and the relatives or friends informed. Transport will be ordered; the general practitioner, health visitor and home nurse will all be informed in good time.

Discharge is frequently preceded by a home visit from the occupational therapist, physiotherapist and/or social worker, to see what problems exist at home. A relative or friend should also be present to give some help and learn what has been decided. The visitor will pay particular attention to the lay-out of the flat or house; whether it is all on the same level or has difficult occasional steps. She will examine the condition of the stairs: whether they are steep; if they have a handrail; whether they are properly lit and whether the stair carpet is worn or frayed. Any loose mats at the top or bottom should be removed. If the patient is unable to go up and down stairs, she will investigate the possibility of bringing the bed downstairs. Many elderly people do not like sleeping downstairs and will be reluctant to agree to this.

The kitchen should also be looked over closely, and the safety of the cooking equipment checked. However, it is no use changing to a more modern appliance if the patient cannot understand its working and has, over many years, become accustomed to using an ancient cooker. If possible, the oven should be table height to avoid bending over and possibly dropping hot dishes and causing burns.

The height of the bed and chair will be noted. The bath too will be inspected; bathing may often prove impossible if the patient lives alone but often it will be found that a special bath seat, bath rails and a non-slip mat on the floor of the bath will enable the patient to manage alone. The lavatory may require appropriate hand rails and the seat may need raising. In many cases there may still be only an outside lavatory and a commode may be needed.

Attention will also be paid to the heating appliances, that they are sufficient in number and are adequately guarded. Many old people still use paraffin heaters as they are an economical form of heating, but they are potentially dangerous. They should be placed in a safe position where they cannot be knocked over and are free from draughts.

Patients who are to live alone after discharge will have been assessed by the occupational therapist on their ability to dress themselves, to cook for themselves, bath, do their washing and all household chores. The patient may be taken to visit the home prior to discharge so that the therapist and social worker may see how the patient reacts and copes with things in his own environment. This is specially useful in the case of the patient who lives alone and who does not wish to leave the sheltered and supportive atmosphere of the hospital and fears loneliness. Once the patient sees his own home again, some enthusiasm returns. On these visits it may be useful for the home nurse or health visitor to be present.

Discharge will never be arranged for a Friday or weekend unless the relatives particularly request it. With few services available over the weekend, it may be disastrous for an elderly person returning to live alone after a spell in hospital to be abandoned for 2 days with no social services.

A home help and meals-on-wheels may have been laid on,

depending on the patient's ability and wishes. Many people like to have them until they find their feet again at home. The home nurse may be asked to call to help with bathing or even dressing, and sometimes to dress an ulcer or give an injection. The health visitor may also be requested to visit to assess whether the patient is managing satisfactorily and to ensure that he is continuing to be mobile and active. Often there is no incentive to be mobile at home and relatives and neighbours are too kind and do too much, leaving the patient to sink back into the condition that existed before treatment.

Case history Mrs X., aged 88 years, lived with a truly devoted husband in a pleasant terraced cottage in the country. She was obese and had gradually become less mobile due to osteoarthritis, and incontinence had resulted. The geratrician visited her and decided that a spell in hospital with intensive rehabilitation was the only possible solution. Progress was slow, impeded by the zealous husband who listened to and sympathized with both parties in the problem, but was always won over by his wife's tears! However, quite good progress was noted and she was eventually discharged home to attend the day hospital regularly to ensure that progress was maintained. However, once she was home, nothing would persuade her to return!

Some of these patients will visit a day centre so that social contact can be maintained and a good meal provided. Even a bath and chiropody service can be obtained.

If the patient is on a special diet, she will have been seen by the dietician and the diet explained with suitable literature given. Relatives too must have the diet and reasons first explained to them. Financial considerations may dictate how far the patient is able to keep to the prescribed diet, and this must be borne in mind.

Drugs at Home

Drugs are a particular problem for the elderly. The patient will have been given a week's supply on discharge from hospital. Drugs should be clearly labelled; the instructions must be explained to the patient, and to the relatives if necessary, and the number reduced to a minimum so that confusion does not occur. Any old drugs accumulated at home should be destroyed where possible to reduce risk of overdosage, wrong dosage or self-administration. So often, elderly people living alone forget to take their drugs and it may be necessary to ask the home nurse or health visitor to call and supervise their administration. The general practitioner will have been informed of the drugs supplied and their dosage so that he can continue their supply and alter the dosage as required.

Some units have a halfway house attached to the rehabilitation ward where the patient can learn to be independent and live with one or two other patients also waiting to go home. Here they can be supervised, assisted and assessed by medical, nursing and therapeutic staff, so that all, including the patient, can be confident that he can manage at home.

Alternative Accommodation

Some patients are no longer able to manage alone in their present accommodation and may require rehousing in a warden-controlled flat where some supervision is available. This change is not normally managed from hospital as there is great demand and long waiting lists for these places. However, the social worker may approach the local housing department, and the patient's name can be placed on the appropriate list.

Others may require housing in residential accommodation for many reasons. The patient may now be too frail physically or unstable mentally to be able to live alone. The relations with whom he may have been living, having enjoyed a period of freedom while their relative was in hospital, are now reluctant to resume their responsibilities. Whatever the reason, the thought of going into a home is regarded with great misgivings by the majority of patients. Loss of independence, personal possessions and a home of their own and, even more, the loss of privacy on entering into a communal life, are thoughts not welcome to elderly persons. Much hard work has to be done by the whole team, specially the nursing staff and social worker who have most opportunity to talk quietly to the patient. The decision should be made slowly; it is not something to be rushed into, and patients should be made to feel that they themselves, and not the hospital authorities or their relatives, have made the decision. Cooperation and support will be sought from the relatives who should also be closely involved in the selection of the home. Choice of a suitable home is all important to the future happiness of the elderly person. An assessment of the patient's income will be made and the value of the patient's house, if there is one, will be properly assessed, as places in local authority homes are few and vacancies in private homes easier to come by. Some people like communal life with plenty of people around; some prefer more seclusion with opportunity to pursue their own hobbies and interests.

There are three categories of old people's homes: local authority, voluntary and private.

Local Authority Homes Residential accommodation provided by the local authority varies from old houses, including old workhouses, converted into homes, to modern purpose-built houses with lifts and other modern devices. The atmosphere, so important to maintain the morale of the residents, will depend almost entirely upon the matron and her staff. The homes are graded as follows:

1. For the physically frail. Grade A for those needing little help or care, Grade B for those needing considerably more care and attention.

2. For the mentally frail; those who are mentally precarious and therefore require much more help on the whole.

Grading is necessary, so that adequate staff can be provided to help the patients. It is important that when application is made for a place in these homes, a true picture of the patient's ability is given, so that he is correctly placed and can receive sufficient help. When an application has been made, a social worker from the community will visit the patient to assess his ability and suitability to enter a home and to ask the patient for his consent for his name to be put forward. They may also discuss the selling of the patient's own property and the disposal of his effects. Many homes do make provision for inmates to take their own ornaments, crockery and a table or chair if they particularly desire this. Meanwhile it is often possible for the social worker or relatives to take the patient to visit a home, so that he can see in advance where he is going. Often the patient is adamant that he does not wish to go, but returns from such a visit with a completely different view of communal life. Before the patient finally goes to a home, he is generally visited by the matron, so that he sees at least one familiar face when he arrives. The home is notified of the approximate time of arrival so that a good welcome can be assured, and it is best if either a relative or social worker can accompany the patient. It is usually best for a patient to go into a home directly from the geriatric unit, so that he has had time for readjustment and has reached his maximum mobility and fitness. If the time spent waiting for a vacancy is too long, the patient can easily deteriorate and no longer qualify for the home proposed.

Voluntary Homes These include convents, Salvation Army homes, Women's Royal Voluntary Service homes, Abbeyfield homes and some homes for those with special needs. Much research is now being done by such associations into the types of homes required by the elderly, and more emphasis is being put on flatlets rather than communal homes. Again careful selection is needed by the social worker for these types of homes. For instance, one would hesitate before suggesting that an atheist or agnostic should go to live in a convent or Salvation Army home, which is obviously appropriate for those who share the convictions of the staff.

Private Homes These vary from guest houses with no nursing care to full-scale nursing homes. These may be better for those who prefer more privacy and less of a communal life. They are generally smaller and often do not enjoy all the amenities of the local authority homes.

Most homes arrange some social activities, often in conjunction with a local school or youth club. The young people may visit and organize communal games. Outings may be possible, visits to local shops and cinemas and even holidays can be arranged. The local clergy may call and hold services or arrange for the inmates to attend local church services. Relatives are normally encouraged to visit as often as possible, and even take the residents out for the day or weekend.

The Out-patient Department

The majority of patients discharged from hospital are followed up in the out-patient department. This is usually not located in the hospital's general out-patient department, where the unsuitable tempo detracts from the value of the appointment. The interview must be leisurely so that the doctor has a chance to examine the patient fully, and is able to listen to any problems that may have arisen. The social worker should be at hand to answer any queries.

The majority of patients are brought in by ambulance and therefore may have some time to wait both before and after appointment.

The Day Hospital

The purpose and functions of a day hospital have already been described in Chapter 2. However its key rôle in the preparation for discharge of a patient must be emphasized here.

A day hospital provides the immediate support and continuity of medical supervision essential in the early days of rehabilitation, which allows discharge from full-time hospital care earlier than would otherwise be possible. Equally important, it allows the transition from hospital back to the outside world to be a gentle one. Most elderly patients have great difficulty in adjusting from the full-time care of the hospital ward to living in their own homes without the 'half-way house' of the day hospital.

Those attending the day hospital will be frequently reviewed in the clinic by the whole team to check that in each case progress is continuing to be made, and that the patient still justifies a place in the hospital. In some cases a case conference will be called involving also the local authority social worker and health visitor, so that future plans can be decided with the whole team, including patient and relatives, present.

Conclusion

The necessity for teamwork in geriatric care is well illustrated by the work of the day hospital, but this is true at every stage of treatment. The whole team work with one objective —the rehabilitation of the patient through the stages of hospital care, to discharge, and to continued care in the community.

While in hospital the patient needs the services of the medical, nursing, therapeutic and social services staff and all the other workers allied to these fields. The nurse's particular rôle is to provide basic nursing care, affording the patient due respect and consideration at all times. Although much of her work is inevitably of a routine and repetitive nature, the nurse has more constant and intimate contact with the patient than any other member of the geriatric team. The success of the patient's stay in hospital will depend upon her patience, understanding and nursing expertise. Thus the value of a well-trained and conscientious geriatric nurse cannot be over-emphasized.

Appendix Equipment in the Geriatric Unit

It would clearly be impractical to attempt to describe all the varieties of equipment which might be found in the geriatric unit, as this will vary considerably from hospital to hospital. However, the nurse in the unit will need to be familiar with the general types of equipment and aids which are available, and should know something about the functioning of at least the most common types.

Beds

King's Fund Bed This is an adjustable height bed, operated by a pump. The head and foot may operate separately. The head is removable and the foot lets down to provide a rack for stripping the bedclothes. The base is solid and a foam mattress is used.

Nesbitt-Evans High–Low Bed The height of this bed is also adjustable, and the head and foot may be elevated separately by means of a lever mechanism.

Bedcradles

Harborough Bedcradle The cradle consists of a strong steel tube, chromium-plated. One end fits under the mattress and the other takes the weight of the bedclothes.

Hoists

Winchester Hoist (Plate X) This is a power-assisted hoist which supports the patient by slings and can thus be alarming when first used. This hoist is fixed in position and can be used either for bathing or for moving the patient in and out of bed.

Ambulift (Plate XI) This lift has a variety of uses, the main purpose being to lift the patient in and out of the bath. It is very stable, as the seat is fixed and there are arm rests, and gives the patient firm security. It can be taken to the bedside and used to help the patient out of bed. The seat can be detached and placed on separate wheels. A bedpan attachment allows it to be used as a commode. If it is necessary to move an exceptionally heavy patient in and out of bed, there are sling attachments, which are very helpful.

Chairs

Many varied geriatric chairs are available, and it is wise to have as large a selection as possible on the ward to accommodate a variety of patients.

Fountain Chair This is a straightforward chair with a back 112 cm (44 in) high and a seat 46 cm (18 in) high. It is vinyl-covered and the arms come well forward.

Tyne Chair This is similar to the Fountain, but has in addition a swivel tray which can be fixed on at a convenient place. The chair may be made mobile by gripping the bars together behind the backrest. This raises the rear chair legs and the whole chair may be pushed forwards.

Easy-to-Rise Chair (Plate XII) This chair is designed for the many old people who find it difficult to rise from an ordinary low chair. The chair legs are splayed out and tipped with rubber to give maximum stability. The angle of the back may be altered and the seat height may be adjusted from 46 cm (18 in) to 60 cm (24 in). The arms project 23 cm (9 in) beyond the front of the seat to provide extra leverage when rising. The covering is washable.

Self-Lift Chair (Plate XIII) This chair has a spring attachment under the seat so that the patient is gently eased up from it. It is useful for patients who have a physical disability which makes it difficult for them to rise initially.

Buxton Chair (Plate XIV) This is another mobile geriatric chair, ideal for the more seriously ill patient who needs greater support. The chair may be tipped backwards through a wide angle, enabling the patient to sleep comfortably if necessary.

Adjustable Lavatory Seats and Frames (Plate XV)

Seat-Aid This is a strong but light steel tube frame which fits round any free-standing lavatory. It has non-slip feet and plastic grips which assist the patient to sit and rise safely.

Plastic Seat-Aid This is a plastic seat which fits directly into the pan and raises the seat by 10 to 15 cm (4 to 6 in).

Adjustable Height Toilet Seat This is a chromium-plated tube frame with moulded plastic arm rests, which enables the seat to be adjusted to the correct height.

Bath Aids

Economic Bath Safety Rail This can be fitted to any bath with conventional taps. Rubber handgrips prevent slipping. It can be moved away above the taps when not not in use.

Projecting Bath Bench and Seat This is designed for those who experience difficulty getting in and out of the bath, owing to weakness or stiffness.

Non-slip Bathmat If placed in the bottom of the bath this reduces the dangers of the patient slipping on the enamel. It is kept in position by rubber suction cups.

Dressing Aids

Lazy Tongs (Plate XVI) These assist dressing generally, and are useful for reaching.

Long-handled Shoehorn (Plate XVII) This is again useful for patients who have difficulty reaching their feet.

Elastic Laces (Plate XVII) These are useful for patients who have to dress using only one hand, or who cannot easily reach their feet.

Stocking Gutter (Plate XVIII) If the patient cannot reach her feet this will be of great assistance in pulling on stockings.

Feeding Aids

Cutlery Handles (Plate XIX) Rubazote sponge tubing is available in 6 gauges for those who have difficulty in gripping narrow handles.

Manoy Cutlery (Plate XX) This is useful for patients who find it difficult to reach their mouths, e.g. in parkinsonism or rheumatoid arthritis.

Nelson Knife (Plate XXI) This knife combines the action of knife and fork; food is cut by a rocking motion on the curve of the blade. It is particularly useful for the hemiplegic patient.

Plate Bunker (Plate XXI) A plastic or Perspex buffer fitted with riveted spring clips which will fit a plate of any reasonable size.

Non-slip Mats (Plate XXI) These mats, which may be made of plastic foam, pimple rubber or plastic webbing, are essential for the disabled.

Manoy Crockery (Plate XX) Melaware make this range of crockery specifically for the disabled.

Walking Aids

Walking Frame (Plate XXII) A frame made of light alloy tubing provides stable but light-weight support between steps for the patient who is mobile but unsteady.

Rollator (Plate XXIII) This frame does not need to be lifted right off the ground between steps, but nor does it run away with the user. It is often useful for those with parkinsonism.

Tripod or Quadriped (Plates XXIV, XXV) Walking sticks with tripod or quadriped bases, made of light-weight tubular steel with rubber feet, give more support than ordinary walking sticks and are useful for the hemiplegic.

Further Reading

Agate, J. (1970) *The Practice of Geriatrics*. London: Heinemann Medical.

Agate, J. (1972) *Geriatrics for Nurses and Social Workers*. London: Heinemann Medical.

Brocklehurst, J. C. (1970) *The Geriatric Day Hospital.*

Bromley, D. B. (1966) *The Psychology of Human Ageing*. Harmondsworth: Penguin.

Felstein, I. (1969) *Later Life: Geriatrics Today and Tomorrow*. Harmondsworth: Penguin.

Ferguson Anderson, W. (1971) *Practical Management of the Elderly*. London: Davis.

Hodkinson, M. (1966) *Nursing the Elderly*. Oxford: Pergamon.

Howell, T. (1970) *A Student's Guide to Geriatrics*. London: Staples.

Irvine, R. E., Bagnall, M. K. & Smith, B. J. (1968) *The Older Patient*. London: English Universities Press.

Isaacs, B. & Livingstone, M. (1972) *Survival of the Unfittest*. London: Routledge and Kegan Paul.

Isaacs, B., Burns, E.M. & Gracie, T. (1973) *Geriatric Nursing*. London: Heinemann Medical.

Rudd, T. N. (1970) *Nursing of the Elderly*. London: Faber.

Townsend, P. (1963) *The Family Life of Old People*. Harmondsworth; Penguin.

Index

The Nurses' Aids Series

NAS

The Nurses' Aids Series is planned to meet the needs of the student nurse during training, and later in qualifying for another part of the Register, by providing a set of textbooks covering most of the subjects included in the general part of the Register and certain specialist subjects. The pupil nurse, too, will find many of these books of particular value and help in practical bedside training. The Series conforms to three factors important to the student:

1. All the authors are nurses who know exactly what the student requires.
2. The books are frequently revised to ensure that advances in knowledge reach the student as soon as practicable.
3. The Aids are well printed and easy to read, clearly illustrated, and modestly priced.

Anaesthesia & Recovery Room Techniques/Wachstein
1976 • 2nd edn.

Anatomy & Physiology for Nurses/Armstrong & Jackson
1972 • 8th edn.

Ear, Nose & Throat Nursing/Marshall & Oxlade *1972 • 5th edn.*

Geriatric Nursing/Storrs
1976 • 1st edn.

A. Medical Nursing/Chapman
1977 • 9th edn.

Microbiology for Nurses/Parker *1978 • 5th edn.*

Obstetric & Gynaecological Nursing/Bailey *1976 • 2nd edn.*

Ophthalmic Nursing/Darling & Thorpe *1975 • 1st edn.*

Orthopaedics for Nurses/ Davies & Stone *1971 • 4th edn.*

Paediatric Nursing/Duncombe & Weller *1974 • 4th edn.*

Personal & Community Health/ Jackson & Lane *1975 • 1st edn.*

Pharmacology for Nurses/ Bailey *1975 • 4th edn.*

Practical Nursing/Clarke *1977 • 12th edn.*

Practical Procedures for Nurses/Billing *1976 • 2nd edn.*

Psychiatric Nursing/Altschul & Simpson *1977 • 5th edn.*

Psychology for Nurses/ Altschul *1975 • 4th edn.*

Sociology for Nurses/Chapman *1978 • 1st edn.*

Surgical Nursing/Fish *1974 • 9th edn.*

Theatre Technique/Houghton & Hudd *1967 • 4th edn.*

NAS Special Interest Texts

See over

For the Advanced Student

NURSES' AIDS SERIES SPECIAL INTEREST TEXTS

Special Interest Texts will enable the student nurse to study a particular subject in greater detail during training or after basic studies have been completed.

Gastroenterological Nursing/ Gribble *1977 • 1st edn.*

Neuromedical & Neurosurgical Nursing/Purchese *1977 • 1st edn.*

Baillière's Medical Transparencies

* A visual reference library for lecturers and students.

*Of special interest to Nurses and Nurse Tutors are 'BMT 1', on the Anatomy of the Head, Neck and Limbs and 'BMT 2', on the Anatomy of the Thorax and Abdomen. Each set illustrates the major anatomical features of the regions with 21 and 18 slides in full colour.

Other sets of interest to nurses specializing in these topics are **Paediatrics** 'BMT 17' and **Venereal Diseases** 'BMT 9' together with **Other Sexually Transmitted Diseases** 'BMT 19'. 24 slides in each set.